THE
MIND
MANUAL

For Shanan, who changed my mind.

An Hachette UK Company
www.hachette.co.uk

First published in Great Britain in 2018 by Hamlyn, a division of
Octopus Publishing Group Ltd
Carmelite House
50 Victoria Embankment
London EC4Y 0DZ
www.octopusbooks.co.uk

Design and Layout Copyright © Octopus Publishing Group Ltd 2018
Text Copyright © Andy Gibson 2018

Distributed in the US by
Hachette Book Group
1290 Avenue of the Americas
4th and 5th Floors
New York, NY 10104

Distributed in Canada by
Canadian Manda Group
664 Annette St.
Toronto, Ontario, Canada M6S 2C8

ISBN 978-0-600-63439-3

A CIP catalogue record for this book is available from the British Library.

Printed and bound in China

10 9 8 7 6 5 4 3 2 1

Publisher: Sarah Ford
Senior Editor: Pollyanna Poulter
Copy Editor: Clare Churly
Senior Designer: Jaz Bahra
Page Layout: Isabel de Cordova
Illustrator: Abigail Read
Senior Production Manager: Peter Hunt

ANDY GIBSON

THE
MIND
MANUAL

mindöpples 5 A DAY FOR A HAPPY, HEALTHY MIND

ABOUT MINDAPPLES

Mindapples is a global campaign that, since 2008, has been teaching people how their minds work and encouraging everyone to take better care of their minds. It builds apps and e-learning, delivers training to businesses and charities, and supplies campaign materials and support to voluntary groups, healthcare bodies, schools and universities to promote mental health and wellbeing.

Its professional training programmes have been used by some of the biggest names in global business, and have been shown in independent trials to help people handle stress and improve their wellbeing. Tens of thousands of people have now shared their 5-a-day for their minds via the Mindapples website, and at events and pop ups all around the world.

www.mindapples.org

@mindapples

ABOUT THE AUTHOR

Andy Gibson is a keynote speaker, author and campaigner specializing in psychology and social change. He is also the founder of several businesses, including Mindapples.

Andy has advised some of the world's biggest businesses on how to harness the minds of their staff, and spent nearly a decade campaigning to raise awareness of the importance of mental health.

His last book, *A Mind for Business*, won Management Gold in the Management Book of the Year awards 2016. He holds degrees in history and psychology, and is also a former Trustee of the Royal Society of Arts. He lives in London.

www.andygibson.org

@gandy

CONTENTS

INTRODUCTION

THIS BOOK ISN'T JUST ABOUT MINDS. THIS BOOK IS ABOUT WHAT IT MEANS TO BE A HUMAN BEING.

The Stoic philosophers of Ancient Rome had a saying: "live according to nature". Whatever you want to do – whether you want to be happy, change the world, make money or be a better person – it's helpful to understand the world, and understand yourself too. The more you know about your mind, and the minds of the people around you, the easier you will find it to get the life you want.

This book is an attempt to share some of what we have learned about the nature of our minds. It is intended as a guide to the odd experiences that each of us have, the moments when our minds do strange things, lead us astray or react in ways we can't explain. It is a book, like so many others before it, about human nature.

A MANUAL FOR THE MIND

Since 2008, Mindapples has been starting positive conversations about looking after our minds, and sharing practical insights to help people improve their lives, work and relationships. It has worked with investment bankers, student nurses, festival-goers, company CEOs, parents, patients, carers and people of all ages and backgrounds, from New York to Sydney, India to Syria.

This book builds on Mindapples' successful "5-a-day for your mind" campaign and training programmes, and shares some of the wisdom that it has gained from talking to thousands of people about their minds. Whatever you're trying to do with your mind, from getting smarter to being kinder, feeling happier or making someone else happy, this book has something to offer.

Its starting point lies in the worlds of psychology and neuroscience. Thanks to new techniques like neuroimaging and cognitive science, we have learned more about the workings of the mind in the last century than we have in the whole of the rest of human history combined. It's time we put this knowledge to the test, to help us make more sense of our minds, and the minds of people around us.

This book is not a synthesis of academic literature though, but an attempt to create something personal and practical, based not on abstract principles but on the insights shared with us through Mindapples' campaign events and training sessions. Our minds are too sensitive and complex to lend themselves to top ten lists or prescription models. Each of us is unique, with different skills and struggles, and we each need to find the things that work best for us.

For all our advances in neuroimaging and experimentation, the human mind remains an elusive subject for study. Neuroscience can tell you which part of your brain feels love, but it can say little about why you miss your family. Science can give us things to think about, but only you know what it is like to be you.

To manage your mind the Mindapples way, you'll need to think about things for yourself. Treat the concepts here as a starting point for a journey of self-discovery, and a chance to reflect on your own experiences. A manual can tell you how a tool works, but it won't tell you what to use it for. What you do with your mind is up to you. As one great amateur psychologist, Bruce Lee, put it, simply take what is useful and develop from there.

WHAT'S GOOD FOR YOUR MIND?

The starting point for our work at Mindapples is always one question: what do you do that's good for your mind? If we can look after our bodies by taking exercise, or eating five fruit and vegetables a day, then what is the equivalent for our minds? The process of learning to manage your mind starts with you. Each of us has a story to tell, and wisdom to offer. This is not a question that can be answered by the experts and mass-produced for everyone: you must play your part. After all, it's your mind.

So alongside the ideas of psychologists and neuroscientists, we've included a completed mindapple at the end of each chapter (see, for example, page 33), to give you an insight into just some of the amazing suggestions people have given us over the years about what they think is good for their minds. Some are wild and crazy, others calm and sensible; some might seem obvious, others you may never have thought about before. Some of them are just downright bonkers. Which is as it should be. The whole point is for you to find your own way, so we have even included some blank mindapples (see pages 9 and 187) for you to fill out yourself. As a wise man once said, we're all individuals. We're all different.

In every country, every community, wherever you are in the world, Mindapples wants to know what works for you. What's the "5-a-day" that's good for your mind? By sharing what works for you, you're adding your wisdom to this conversation about what we need to feel happy and healthy, and hopefully inspiring others to share what works for them too. Through this, and through the many other ideas and questions explored in this book, we hope to start conversations all around the world about what each of us needs to feel good, get along and enjoy our lives.

Of course, a book like this can only scratch the surface of such a complex topic, but, hopefully, it will help you appreciate your mind a little more, and perhaps inspire you to get people talking about what their minds need and how we can all live and work better. It's a chance for you to explore your mind, think about what it needs, and perhaps feel a bit more compassion for yourself and others.

So let's start by exploring what it means to be you, and what you need to know about yourself in order to get the life you want. What's it like inside your mind?

KNOW YOUR MIND

mindapples

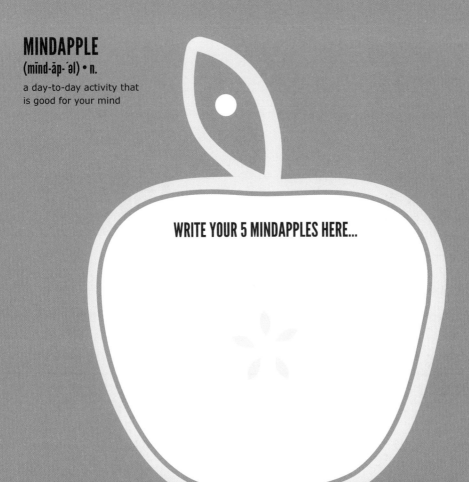

MINDAPPLE

(mīnd-āp-´əl) • n.

a day-to-day activity that
is good for your mind

WRITE YOUR 5 MINDAPPLES HERE...

You will see mindapples throughout this book. Some have been filled in using responses from the Mindapples community; some – like this one – are blank. Why not take a moment now to fill in your first mindapple?

Think about your mind. What works for you?
What calms you down, wakes you up or makes you happy?
What's the 5-a-day for your mind?

Write down five things you do that are good for your mind.
We'll come back to this at the end of the book...

HOW
TO
BE
YOURSELF

HOW TO BE YOURSELF

"JUST BE YOURSELF"

Whether you've been nervous about a job interview, preparing for a first date, or just worrying about life in general, somebody has probably told you to "be yourself".

It's hard to know how to take this. After all, who else would you be? Like it or not, we are stuck with ourselves. So is it possible you aren't being yourself? How can you tell when you are being you, and when you aren't? Which one is the real you?

From the four humours to horoscopes, the study of what makes each of us unique goes back centuries. Modern psychologists continue to wrestle with this challenge today. A 2015 study conducted at the University of Houston identified four factors that can help you be "true to yourself":

- **SELF-AWARENESS:** Being curious about yourself, and aware of who you are, what you're doing, and why you're doing it.
- **OBJECTIVITY:** Being unbiased in your thoughts, and accepting the truth about yourself.
- **CONSISTENCY:** Doing what you say, and living according to your own values and principles rather than those of others.
- **HONESTY:** Being able to be yourself and express your needs in the company of others, particularly in close relationships.

So let's begin at the beginning. In order to be yourself, first you have to know yourself. What's your comfort zone? What are your strengths and weaknesses? Where do you feel at home? To answer these questions, you need to understand your mind, know how it works, and what makes it unique. To get the life that's right for you, you need to know who you are, and what you need – or else you could end up with someone else's perfect life.

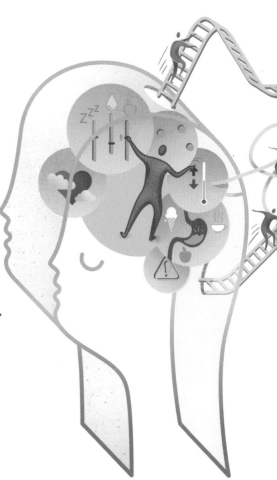

IN TWO MINDS

Have you ever done something, and then wondered why you did it? One of the strangest things about being human is that often we do things we didn't mean to do. You eat cake when you're on a diet, shout at someone when you're stressed, stay up late when you need an early night. Sometimes it can feel like your mind is running your life for you. So how can this be? Which of these impulses is the *real* you?

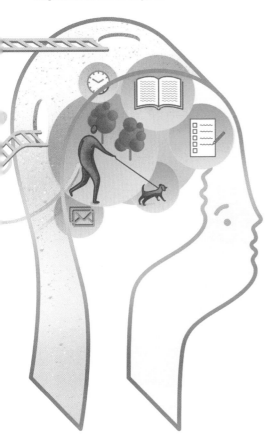

Philosophers have wrestled with this conflict for centuries. Classical Greek philosophers talked about reason and appetite, and Christian theologians spoke of grace and sin. Then, in the 19th century, the psychoanalyst Sigmund Freud and his contemporaries developed one of the most important ideas in psychology: the unconscious mind. The unconscious was first thought to be a place of dark secrets and wild desires, but modern psychologists see the unconscious rather differently. Unconscious mental processes are simply those that you can't identify and control, and which happen without your choosing.

Most of what happens in your unconscious is actually quite dull. It digests food for you, lets you know when you're feeling cold, alerts you to potential dangers, remembers your PIN number, and so on. Beneath your conscious thoughts, your mind keeps track of everything for you, from the tingle in your fingers to the heartbeat that keeps them warm, or the nagging doubt that you've left the iron on. Your unconscious is like a helpful assistant, handling all the boring things and leaving your conscious mind free to think about more important matters.

So when it comes to knowing yourself, your conscious thoughts are just the tip of the iceberg. To really know yourself, you need to look a bit deeper.

THE SPRINTER AND THE THINKER

Perhaps the best model we've found so far for making sense of the divided nature of the self is dual process theory, a model of the mind championed by pioneers such as the Nobel prize-winning psychologist, Daniel Kahneman. Dual process theory argues that we have two distinct types of thought: a first, quick, instinctive response and a second, slower, thoughtful response.

Writers have given many names to these two responses over the years. Social psychologist Jonathan Haidt in *The Happiness Hypothesis* calls them the elephant and the rider; psychiatrist Steve Peters in *The Chimp Paradox* calls them the chimp and the human; Daniel Kahneman in *Thinking, Fast and Slow* calls them System 1 and System 2. In this book we will call them the sprinter and the thinker.

These two responses aren't separate; they are just two different thought processes that you use every day, and they work together. They are both you. The unifying idea at the heart of dual process theory is that your mind is best understood as two types of thinking operating in tandem.

THE SPRINTER

Your first response, the sprinter, leaps into the action quickly, reacting to your environment, always eager to help. It offers up basic reactions, such as a desire to approach or run away, feelings of fear, anger or curiosity, and connections to memories, associations and past experiences.

The sprinter evolved to navigate day-to-day life, watching your surroundings, spotting opportunities and reacting to threats. Some of its responses seem to be in-built, such as stress or hunger, but others develop from experience, as your mind learns to deal with common situations.

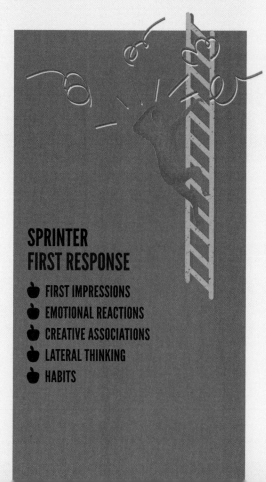

SPRINTER FIRST RESPONSE

- 👆 FIRST IMPRESSIONS
- 👆 EMOTIONAL REACTIONS
- 👆 CREATIVE ASSOCIATIONS
- 👆 LATERAL THINKING
- 👆 HABITS

From learning your times tables to remembering your friends' faces, the sprinter is the key to getting through each day. Without it, you wouldn't be reading this book; you'd still be lying in bed trying to figure out how to get up.

THE THINKER

Your first response is essential, but it isn't always reliable, because many of the habits and associations your mind learns are wrong. You have lots of responses flashing through your mind, but you wouldn't want to act on all of them. For this reason, you have also evolved a second response, the thinker, which you use when you put your conscious attention on something and think it through.

The thinker in you considers things more deeply, breaking down situations carefully and following logical processes rather than free associations. It is capable of complex analytic tasks such as logical thought or mental arithmetic – but it is slower than the sprinter. To work well, your thinker needs time to concentrate.

The thinker also requires more energy. Your sprinter is very economical in how it uses resources, so it can operate for a long time without running out of steam. Your thinker is more demanding. Thinking things through takes effort. It's a form of physical work and it can tire you out. The more you use your conscious mind, the harder it gets to think things through until you stop to rest.

No wonder, then, that only a fraction of your behaviour is driven by your conscious mind. Most of what you do during the day is instinctive, handled automatically by your first response without you thinking about it at all. You simply don't have the time, or the energy, to think everything through.

THINKER
SECOND RESPONSE

- SECOND THOUGHTS
- ANALYTIC THINKING
- FOCUSED ATTENTION
- PROBLEM-SOLVING
- THOUGHTS

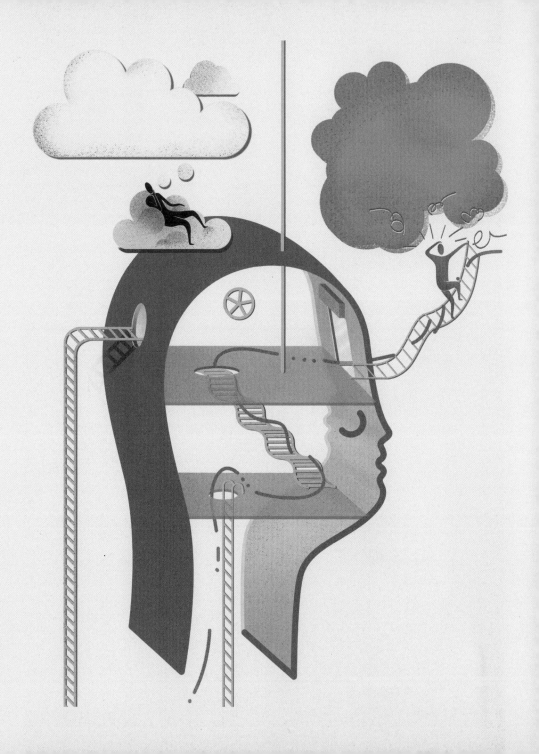

FIND YOUR MIND

mindapples

KNOW YOUR MIND

To know yourself, you have to understand your first response, learn what it needs and be aware of what it's likely to do next. You need to know what your mind gets up to when you're not paying attention.

HOW WELL DO YOU KNOW YOURSELF?

Most of us like to think we know ourselves pretty well. After all, we spend our lives inside our heads, so we should know something about what we want and need by now. But how sure can you be of how you'll react in a given situation? For example, how do you react to uncertainty? Do you find it exciting or frightening? What's your attitude to learning? Do you enjoy it or find it tiring? Do you cope well with arguments and conflict or find them upsetting? Do you find other people energizing or get tired in company? Do you need to plan ahead or would you rather just go with the flow?

It can be hard to step back and see yourself in an honest, objective way

Questions such as these can seem simple, but unravelling them can take a lifetime. For one thing, it's hard to look at yourself objectively. Most of us – particularly men – tend to overestimate our abilities and imagine ourselves to be braver, smarter and stronger than we are, so being told the truth about yourself can be a blow to your self-image.

We also get confusing feedback from the people around us. Friends may tell us nice things to spare our feelings, and bullies may criticize us unfairly. Getting accurate information is difficult, and we often have no standard against which to compare it, because we never really know what other people are like. Faced with all this, it can be hard to step back and see yourself in an honest, objective way.

PERSONALITY PSYCHOLOGY

This is where personality psychology can help. The study of personality is the study of what makes each of us unique. There have been many decades of research on personality, and although it is necessarily a complex area to research, some helpful patterns are emerging. Understanding your personality is a good start for understanding yourself.

THE BIG FIVE

1. **EXTROVERSION**
2. **SENSITIVITY**
3. **CONSCIENTIOUSNESS**
4. **AGREEABLENESS**
5. **OPENNESS**

FIVE TRAITS, MANY COMBINATIONS

The most widely used model of personality in modern psychology is the Big Five, which maps our personalities on five scales or traits. **Each trait describes a different aspect of your personality, and you can be strong or weak in each trait, creating thousands of possible combinations.**

Every one of the traits is healthy and normal, so the main lesson from the Big Five is just how much natural variation there is between us. We are a complicated and unpredictable bunch, but the model can help you figure out

more precisely how you differ from other people, and what you need.

Over the following pages you'll learn about the five traits. Don't try to look at them all together yet: start by trying to understand where you are in relation to each individual trait, and then look at all the traits together to build a picture of who you are.

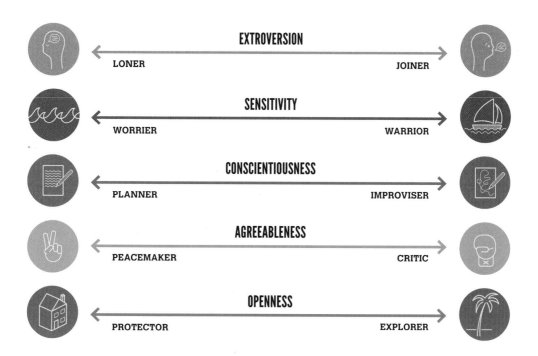

EXTROVERSION

LONER — JOINER

SENSITIVITY

WORRIER — WARRIOR

CONSCIENTIOUSNESS

PLANNER — IMPROVISER

AGREEABLENESS

PEACEMAKER — CRITIC

OPENNESS

PROTECTOR — EXPLORER

LONERS AND JOINERS

The first trait in the Big Five is extroversion. People who are high in this trait enjoy external rewards and social interactions, possibly because their brains respond more strongly to external rewards. People lower in this trait are described as introverted, which is a tendency to focus on inner satisfaction, thoughts and ideas rather than the world around you.

This isn't about being good with people – introverts can be very socially skilled, and extroverts can struggle in relationships – this is about where you get your energy. If you find yourself sitting at home thinking, "I should go out and see people; that will wake me up," you're probably more of an extrovert. If you're out with friends, thinking, "I love my friends but I need to go home and read my book or I'll be exhausted tomorrow," you're probably more of an introvert.

How high or low do you think you are in extroversion? Which sounds more like you?

There's no right or wrong answer. Being introverted or extroverted are both natural and normal. Just think about what you prefer, and what you enjoy. If you are more introverted, you will enjoy your own company and need less attention from people around you – but you can still go out with your friends and have great relationships. If you're more of an extrovert, you can still be on your own or listen quietly

to people, but you might prefer going out more and love talking to people. Everyone has their own comfort zone.

Most of us are somewhere in the middle. Although some people are extremely introverted or extroverted, this isn't about categorizing people into types. If you display

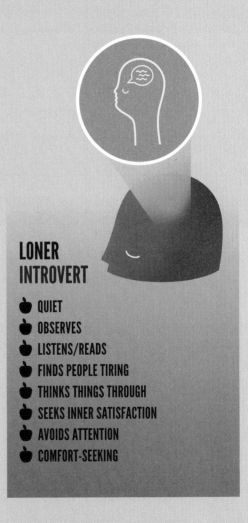

LONER INTROVERT

- 👍 QUIET
- 👍 OBSERVES
- 👍 LISTENS/READS
- 👍 FINDS PEOPLE TIRING
- 👍 THINKS THINGS THROUGH
- 👍 SEEKS INNER SATISFACTION
- 👍 AVOIDS ATTENTION
- 👍 COMFORT-SEEKING

some characteristics from each, you're probably around 50 percent in the trait of extroversion. Some people might describe you as an "ambivert".

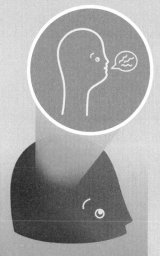

JOINER EXTROVERT

- 🍎 LOUD
- 🍎 PARTICIPATES
- 🍎 TALKS/DISCUSSES
- 🍎 FINDS PEOPLE ENERGIZING
- 🍎 TALKS THINGS THROUGH
- 🍎 SEEKS EXTERNAL PLEASURES
- 🍎 ENJOYS ATTENTION
- 🍎 THRILL-SEEKING

MANAGING EXTROVERSION

There's nothing wrong with being introverted or extroverted, but both may need to be managed.

If you're very introverted, you might need to push yourself to spend time with people, even though you find it tiring. If you're very extroverted, you might need to make an effort to keep quiet and not dominate social situations. And that's fine. Remember, just because you have a first response to talk, or to keep quiet, you can still choose to act differently. Think about the situation you're in, and the way you want it to go, and manage your first response accordingly.

Extroverts do seem to be a little happier though, on average at least, and this might be because we tend to overlook introverts and give more opportunities to louder people. In her book *Quiet*, Susan Cain makes a compelling case for why introverts are valuable and needed, and why we need to make more effort to harness their skills, particularly in work.

So if you are an introvert, don't try to change yourself, because you have a lot to offer, but you might want to push yourself forward from time to time to make sure you aren't ignored. And if you're an extrovert, try to make sure you don't overlook the quiet people in your enthusiasm for life.

WORRIERS AND WARRIORS

The next trait in the Big Five is sensitivity, more technically known as neuroticism. This trait describes how responsive you are to negative situations, such as threats and criticism. People who are high in sensitivity will tend to feel bad things more deeply, in the same way that a strong response to good things is more associated with extroversion.

Being sensitive to negative responses will tend to make you more cautious, as you naturally want to prevent things going wrong. In extreme forms, this can be a burden, and people with higher sensitivity tend to be more at risk of depression and anxiety, but it's perfectly possible to be sensitive and have a good life. In fact, this trait can be associated with pushing yourself and seeking achievement, rather than being satisfied with less. People lower in this trait, though, can handle setbacks better and are less stressed by everyday life – even if everyone has their breaking point.

How high or low do you think you are in sensitivity? Which sounds more like you?

There's nothing wrong with being very sensitive, or being very resilient: each is useful in different situations. Wherever you are on the scale, it's worth thinking about your sensitivity, and the sensitivities of the people around you.

People who are highly sensitive can still feel calm and happy, but they might need to manage their moods and way of life more to stay comfortable. Someone who's lower in sensitivity may be able to bounce back more quickly from setbacks, but they will still get stressed and feel sad at times.

It's not always comfortable being sensitive, and it can be tempting to envy people who

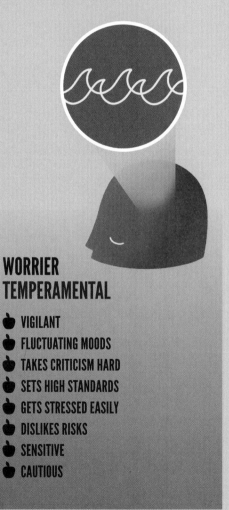

WORRIER
TEMPERAMENTAL

- VIGILANT
- FLUCTUATING MOODS
- TAKES CRITICISM HARD
- SETS HIGH STANDARDS
- GETS STRESSED EASILY
- DISLIKES RISKS
- SENSITIVE
- CAUTIOUS

are more robust and those who can shake off criticism and bounce back quickly from problems. However, this trait has been very important over the centuries, both for inspiring people to make the world safer, and for encouraging empathy for other people who feel bad, and helping them to recover.

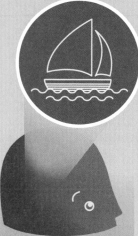

WARRIOR
EVEN-TEMPERED

- 🍎 RELAXED
- 🍎 STABLE MOODS
- 🍎 SHRUGS OFF CRITICISM
- 🍎 ACCEPTS FLAWS AND FAILURES
- 🍎 GETS STRESSED RARELY
- 🍎 TOLERATES RISKS
- 🍎 RESILIENT
- 🍎 CAREFREE

MANAGING SENSITIVITY

There's no way around it: sensitive people will need to manage their moods and habits more carefully than their less sensitive peers. Being sensitive to threats means you're cautious – because you will feel things more deeply than the people around you – so you may have to stick up for yourself when people are pushing you out of your comfort zone. Take note of the situations where you feel safe, and try to push yourself to take risks, but be kind when you need to stop. You might also have to remind yourself that people aren't trying to upset you; they just see the world differently.

If you're lower in sensitivity, you may find all this business of managing moods and thinking about your mind a bit boring: life is good so why worry? So you may need to force yourself to see things from other people's perspectives and not be too quick to judge when someone is upset or scared. Think about how you feel doing something that really scares you, such as public speaking, and remember some people feel that way just going to a party or meeting your parents.

Although all the Big Five traits are separate, they will interact. If you're high in extroversion, this will make you very sensitive to positive and negative events, meaning life can feel like an emotional rollercoaster. Many outgoing people struggle with their emotions behind closed doors. Conversely, sensitive introverts may be shy and avoid people altogether.

PLANNERS AND IMPROVISERS

The third trait is conscientiousness, which is linked to your capacity to control your behaviour and work toward long-term goals.

People high in conscientiousness have good attention to detail and a strong sense of how the world should be. They make a lot of plans, they are more likely to keep their promises, and they are also more likely to live according to their principles, such as by being vegetarian. People who are high in this trait tend to find it easier to stick with their decisions and persist at difficult tasks. Practising skills, resisting temptation, being organized, all come more naturally to someone high in conscientiousness. In extreme forms, though, they may struggle with change and be too rigid in their thinking, missing out on opportunities and finding it hard to cope with the messiness of life.

People who are low in conscientiousness can still plan ahead, but it doesn't come naturally to them, and so they have to make more effort to follow through on their intentions. If your motto is "Let's see what happens," you may be lower in conscientiousness. If you find yourself shouting, "Just tell me the plan!" then you may be higher in this trait.

How high or low do you think you are in conscientiousness? Which sounds more like you?

Since conscientiousness is associated with high standards and increased willpower, it's one of the more sought-after traits. Being

able to control your impulses and work to long-term goals is advantageous in education, career development, relationships and self-management, so it is a good predictor of long-term success in life and work.

People who are low in conscientiousness may struggle to stick to plans and work toward

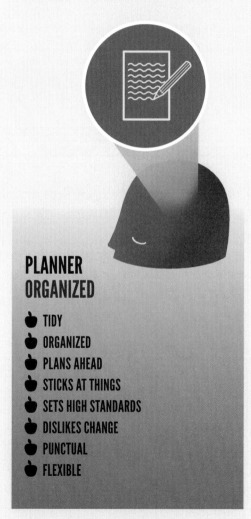

PLANNER
ORGANIZED

- 🍎 TIDY
- 🍎 ORGANIZED
- 🍎 PLANS AHEAD
- 🍎 STICKS AT THINGS
- 🍎 SETS HIGH STANDARDS
- 🍎 DISLIKES CHANGE
- 🍎 PUNCTUAL
- 🍎 FLEXIBLE

goals, but they may be better at coping with uncertainty, going with the flow and tolerating the flaws of other people. Again, there's no right or wrong way to be. Planning is important, but in uncertain times, when plans keep going wrong, it can be helpful to have people around who enjoy the chaos and can cope with uncertainty.

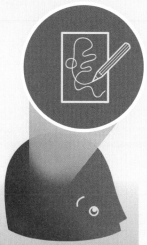

IMPROVISER
DISORGANIZED

- 👎 UNTIDY
- 👎 DISORGANIZED
- 👎 GOES WITH THE FLOW
- 👎 EASILY DISTRACTED
- 👎 ACCEPTS THINGS AS THEY ARE
- 👎 HANDLES CHANGE WELL
- 👎 SPONTANEOUS
- 👎 RELIABLE

MANAGING CONSCIENTIOUSNESS

If you're lower in conscientiousness, you may struggle to do what you intended to do, so it's worth managing yourself more closely. You may need more support with sticking to decisions and working toward goals. People who are very low in conscientiousness may even struggle with addictions or getting qualifications. If you can find a job you love, and good supportive relationships, you may find planning for the future gets easier.

If you're high in conscientiousness, you may have the opposite problem, of being too rigid and missing out on opportunities because they don't fit with the plan. It may feel like the world doesn't live up to your standards, and you may find the chaos and messiness of other people a bit maddening. Try to remember that while plans are great, you can't control everything – and sometimes, chaos can even be fun.

If you're quite introverted and conscientious, you may enjoy solitary pursuits, jobs that involve attention to detail and working on your own. If you're an extrovert, you may find yourself trying to control conversations and organize everyone around you, so remember to leave space for other people to be heard and let them do what they want.

Being highly conscientious doesn't have to mean you find chaos upsetting – you just enjoy order more – but if you're high in sensitivity, you may end up being a bit of a perfectionist, setting high standards and never being satisfied with what you've achieved. You may also find change upsetting, and other people's insensitivity or risk-taking distressing.

PEACEMAKERS AND CRITICS

The fourth trait is agreeableness. In literal terms, this is about your willingness to agree, but a more fitting description of this trait might be a desire for harmony.

Your level of agreeableness describes your natural level of empathy and consideration for others, and your concern for how other people think and feel. People who are high in agreeableness tend to be generous, trusting and forgiving, concerned for others and distressed by conflict. People who are lower in this trait cope better with arguments, find it easier to be critical and are less worried when people don't get along or don't like them.

People who are high in agreeableness can still have arguments, and people who are low in it can still be nice. This is just about whether upsetting people makes you uncomfortable, and if you will prioritize keeping the peace over things that matter to you. If you find yourself saying, "I know you're upset but we need to get it right," you may be lower in agreeableness; if you keep saying, "Whatever you want to do," you may be higher in agreeableness.

How high or low do you think you are in agreeableness? Which sounds more like you?

We tend to prefer spending time with agreeable people as they tolerate our weaknesses and tend to be trustworthy and helpful.

Since agreeableness is associated with some very positive, likeable traits, you might expect this to be a trait everyone wants to have. In reality, though, people often look down on highly agreeable people because they can be seen as a bit of a pushover and lacking in critical faculties.

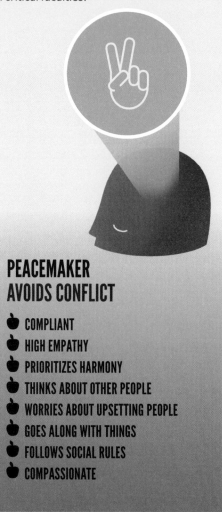

PEACEMAKER AVOIDS CONFLICT

- COMPLIANT
- HIGH EMPATHY
- PRIORITIZES HARMONY
- THINKS ABOUT OTHER PEOPLE
- WORRIES ABOUT UPSETTING PEOPLE
- GOES ALONG WITH THINGS
- FOLLOWS SOCIAL RULES
- COMPASSIONATE

People lower in this trait may upset people and find themselves in frequent arguments and disputes, which can be exhausting for the people around them. In some situations, particularly high-pressure work environments, it can be an advantage to be disagreeable as it may be seen as assertiveness and ambition.

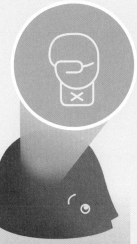

CRITIC
ENJOYS CONFLICT

- CRITICAL
- LOW EMPATHY
- PRIORITIZES QUALITY
- THINKS ABOUT SELF
- DOESN'T MIND UPSETTING PEOPLE
- GOES AGAINST THE GRAIN
- IGNORES SOCIAL RULES
- INDIFFERENT

MANAGING AGREEABLENESS

High agreeableness is generally an advantage in life, since it brings with it lower stress levels, better relationships and overall life satisfaction. Putting other people first really does seem to work as a strategy for life.

The problems may come in work situations, or other environments where you need to push yourself forward or fight for what you want. Agreeable people get jobs more easily and tend to stay in work, but they often struggle to get promoted, and there are many cases of people having to learn to be more disagreeable to get ahead and catch people's attention.

This trait can clash with conscientiousness: if you have a strong sense of how things should be, this can bring you into conflict with people, and you may have to choose between peace and principles. Less agreeable people might be more willing to upset people in order to get things exactly right.

This trait and extroversion have the most influence on your relationships: disagreeable extroverts may be domineering and difficult, while agreeable introverts may be overlooked easily and struggle to make an impression. High agreeableness is generally an advantage for both sides though.

If you're high in sensitivity and agreeableness, you may be particularly worried about what people think about you and be nervous in groups. This sort of social anxiety can become a burden, and can make it particularly hard to be honest about how you feel and be true to yourself in company.

PROTECTORS AND EXPLORERS

The final trait in the Big Five is openness to experience. This trait describes how you process information and take on new ideas, and is linked to creativity and open-mindedness.

People who are high in openness are curious about the world and enjoy new information and experiences, such as travel and learning. They may have a wide range of interests and are excited by new things. They may also enjoy creative pursuits such as art and literature, and be original in their thinking.

People lower in this trait prefer familiarity to novelty, and are more naturally conservative. They know what they like and dislike change. They may also be better at appreciating what they have, upholding traditions and preserving what works. If you prefer familiar situations and dislike change, you're probably lower in openness. If you get bored as soon as you've figured out how to do something, you're probably higher.

How high or low do you think you are in openness? Which sounds more like you?

If you're the sort of person who reads books about how the mind works, then the chances are you are higher in this trait than the average person. Openness is just one end of the spectrum though. For many of us, novelty is not to be welcomed, but to be viewed with caution.

Openness is linked to pattern recognition and intelligence, so it can be a big advantage in a world where the sheer volume of information facing us is overwhelming. People who are low in openness may be unwilling to question their core beliefs, and can be more prone to bias and prejudice. People very high in openness may be

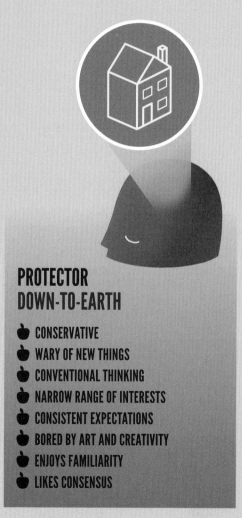

PROTECTOR
DOWN-TO-EARTH

- CONSERVATIVE
- WARY OF NEW THINGS
- CONVENTIONAL THINKING
- NARROW RANGE OF INTERESTS
- CONSISTENT EXPECTATIONS
- BORED BY ART AND CREATIVITY
- ENJOYS FAMILIARITY
- LIKES CONSENSUS

too quick to take silly ideas seriously though, and unable to stick at things and see them through.

As with all the Big Five traits, there isn't a "right way" to be. It's about knowing yourself well enough to manage your weaknesses, play to your strengths, and seek out the situations that suit you best.

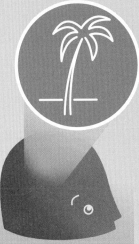

EXPLORER
ADVENTUROUS

- 🍎 CREATIVE
- 🍎 LIKES NEW THINGS
- 🍎 UNUSUAL THINKING
- 🍎 WIDE RANGE OF INTERESTS
- 🍎 UNEXPECTED ASSOCIATIONS
- 🍎 INTERESTED IN ART AND CREATIVITY
- 🍎 ENJOYS NOVELTY
- 🍎 LIKES DIVERSITY

MANAGING OPENNESS

If you are high in openness, your main enemy will be boredom. People high in this trait find it hard to do repetitive tasks and need constant novelty. Sticking to plans and doing easy tasks may feel frustrating, and you might need to make more of an effort to do things once you've mastered them.

People lower in this trait may tend to be conservative and wary of change, and so may have to work harder to keep up with new ideas and avoid being left behind. If you're low in this trait, you may have to force yourself to keep an open mind, and spot when your resistance to change becomes irrational.

The drive to try new things can be a distraction from getting things done, particularly if you're also low in conscientiousness.

If you're high in extroversion and in openness, you might spend all your time meeting new people but struggle to form lasting relationships. If you're low in openness, you may take risky or unwise decisions in pursuit of rewards, and be unwilling to hear criticism or question your thinking.

If you are high in sensitivity, high openness may lead you to seek out new experiences even though you find them stressful and upsetting, and you may need to resist the urge to smash up your comfortable life.

If you're low in agreeableness and high in openness, you may well enjoy debates and arguments that other people find distressing or pointless. Seek out people who disagree with you, but remember to argue gently.

WHO ARE YOU?

So where do you think you fall on the personality map? You can get some idea of your personality by listing some of the traits outlined on the previous pages that you think apply to you (there is a Notes section starting on page 182 that you can use to do just that), or by taking a Big Five personality test free online. Don't take such tests too seriously though: unless you're paying for a professional one, it's only really a guide. The important thing is to reflect on your behaviour, and think about how you react in different situations. Self-awareness isn't a scientific process: it can take years to figure out who you are – and even then, you may still surprise yourself.

Your personality can't explain you entirely, of course. Your personality traits just describe what comes naturally to you, your sensitivities and tendencies, and the patterns of how you think, feel and react. You also have your habits, the conditioning and learned responses that you've built up over time to handle everything that comes at you. And you have the experiences and memories you've gained over your life, and your upbringing and culture, all of which change how you see the world and react to situations.

Your personality traits say nothing about your hobbies, sexual preferences, cultural attitudes, beliefs, dress sense or values. Someone who shares your personality traits, but who was born two hundred years ago, would not be the same as you. They'd have different memories and cultural associations,

and different strategies for dealing with the world. However, if you were ever to meet them, you might notice some uncanny similarities in how you both react to situations.

Understanding your personality isn't the only way to know yourself, but it's a great place to start. Comprehending the basic patterns in how you feel and how you react can help you understand why you react differently to people around you, and what you need to feel happy and comfortable.

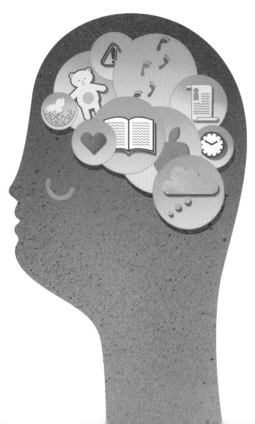

CHANGING YOUR MIND

It may be that you don't like your personality, or at least some aspects of it. You may even be tempted to act differently, put on a mask and pretend to be someone else. In fact, playing with new roles and trying new behaviours can be a fantastic way to learn about yourself.

BUT CAN YOU REALLY CHANGE?
Your personality is at least partly genetic, the result of your physiology and consequently hard to change, rather like changing your height. However, a large part of who you are is affected by your culture, upbringing and life choices, just as a germinating seed is affected by the water and sunlight it receives. In fact, with the emerging field of epigenetics, some aspects of your genetic code may even be shaped by your environment and upbringing.

Personality traits describe the long-term trends in your behaviour, so by definition, changing your personality takes a long time. Yet it can be done. Significant life events can shift your personality, and people tend to become more conscientious, introverted and resilient as they grow older. Stable relationships and a job you love can also help you feel less sensitive and more conscientious, and new experiences can increase your openness.

You can also consciously shift your personality traits by pushing yourself out of your comfort zone, training yourself to go against your natural instincts. If you don't enjoy socializing but know you need to make friends, you can still act in a more extroverted way.

Just be aware that constantly reminding yourself to act differently is more tiring than just acting on instinct. Being yourself is always easier than acting like someone else.

Changing your personality takes a long time. Yet it can be done

Your personality is not a prison though. Your first response (see page 14) doesn't define you, and being yourself doesn't mean being a slave to your instincts. It means knowing yourself well enough to anticipate your reactions, and manage yourself accordingly. Your personality helps you predict what your first response might be, but you are always free to have second thoughts.

BEING YOURSELF

Being yourself, then, is perhaps best understood as doing what's most comfortable for you. That doesn't mean you have to stop pushing yourself to try new things, or caring about other people's needs, but it does mean living and reacting in a way that comes naturally to you.

Part of this is about being honest with other people about how you feel, and not feeling you need to suppress part of yourself or pretend to be something you're not. Again, your personality traits can help you get better at this.

- If you're high in agreeableness, you may struggle to ask for what you need. Experiment with telling people how you feel, and find ways of talking about what you need without feeling pushy or needy. If you care about other people's feelings, then it's OK to care about your own feelings too.
- If you're very sensitive, you may need to be careful with yourself. Avoid stress and watch out for beating yourself up or taking criticism too hard.
- If you're low in conscientiousness, you may struggle to behave in a way that's consistent with your values. Try to be honest with yourself and accept your failings, rather than holding yourself to impossible standards.
- If you're very extrovert, try not to lose yourself in other people, or in the constant search for praise. Make time for quiet reflection and try to spend a bit of time alone.
- If you're high in openness, make sure that your quest for knowledge and experiences

doesn't leave you adrift with no position of your own. Sometimes it's important to stick with things and preserve what works.

Despite how simple it sounds, there's a lot involved in being yourself. Being yourself takes courage: it may not come easily to you to ask for what you need and be yourself in all situations. Being yourself isn't a burden though: you are always free to be someone else for a while. Just learn where you feel comfortable, so that when you need to, you can find your way home.

Don't spend your life pretending to be someone you're not. It's far better to be a good version of yourself than a bad version of someone else. The purpose of your life is yours to choose, so learn who you are and what you want, so that you end up with your perfect life, and not the one you were told to want.

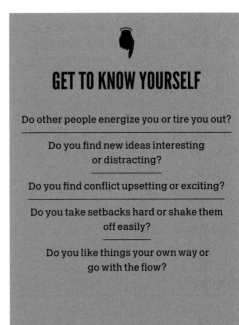

GET TO KNOW YOURSELF

Do other people energize you or tire you out?

Do you find new ideas interesting or distracting?

Do you find conflict upsetting or exciting?

Do you take setbacks hard or shake them off easily?

Do you like things your own way or go with the flow?

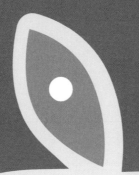

WHAT WORKS FOR YOU?

Look through old travel photos.

Talk to my parents on the phone.

Listen to my favourite music.

Remind myself that I am good enough.

Onion gravy on everything.

HOW TO KEEP CALM

YOUR EMOTIONAL MIND

There is a 14th-century philosophical joke about a logical donkey. Affectionately named Buridan's ass, after the French philosopher Jean Buridan, this unfortunate animal is placed equidistant between two identical piles of food – and starves to death. With no reason to pick one pile of food over the other, the donkey refuses to choose.

Such humour may be an acquired taste, but the example illustrates the limitations of logic. The sensible thing for the donkey to do is to eat any pile at random, but without a reason to act, it does nothing.

We may like to think of ourselves as calm and rational people, planning ahead and arguing our case, but in reality we live much more emotionally. We feel sad about the past, worry about the future and get angry when someone gets in our way. Whether we admit it or not, each and every one of us is emotional.

In fact, people whose emotional systems have been damaged can experience the problem of Buridan's ass in real life. They may not worry as much about the future, but give them a simple choice such as what to eat for lunch, and they can't choose. Without emotions, we struggle to take action.

THE POWER OF EMOTIONS

Although it might not feel like it some of the time, emotions are actually pretty useful.

They change how you see the world and give you information about how to respond to events. Your mind is constantly scanning your environment for threats and opportunities, but there is too much information to process consciously, so instead your mind filters it through your emotions. They are your mind's way of calling your attention to what matters, and spotting what's important.

Negative emotions such as fear and anger focus your mind on problems, signalling that there is something you need to do. They narrow your focus and limit your options to help you take quick, decisive action to improve your situation. Unfortunately they can also make you miss opportunities and pay too much attention to negative events and bad memories.

On the other hand, positive emotions such as joy and excitement are signals that it is safe to explore and pursue opportunities. When you are in a positive state of mind, you literally see more around you. (There's more on this in the next chapter.)

MANAGING YOUR EMOTIONS

Your feelings are always there and you can't switch them off. All you can do is manage them, by keeping an eye on how they are

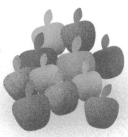

affecting your thoughts and behaviour, and taking steps to deal with them. How well you control your emotions determines whether they end up helping you, or ruling you. Keeping calm isn't just a matter of feeling good, it's also a crucial part of leading a happy, successful life.

There are lots of different emotional states, each subtly different, but the two that most affect our ability to keep calm are fear and anger. Both emotions are useful, but both can take over your mind and cause you to overreact, make mistakes and create problems – angry people take stupid risks, while fearful people miss opportunities. Managing these two feelings is the starting point for keeping calm.

It isn't always possible to think your way through a problem. Sometimes there genuinely isn't a clear reason to do one thing or another, and the choice to act is emotional instead. You have to feel your way to the right decision.

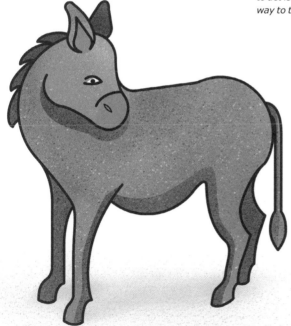

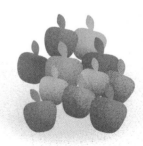

STRESS

One of the biggest barriers to staying calm is stress. Stress is a fear response, a sign that you feel like you are in danger. It is a natural part of being human, and not a disease or a weakness.

Stress is a legacy from our evolutionary past, and it's adapted perfectly for dealing with the primal threats that faced our ancestors thousands of years ago.

For example, let's imagine that a sabre-toothed tiger is attacking you. The stress response kicks in, your mind focuses on the tiger, your heart beats faster, cortisol rushes around your system and you have the energy you need to fight the tiger or run away from the tiger – the famous fight-or-flight response.

You wouldn't want to lose your stress response because it's useful to react quickly to danger. Take away your stress response and you might feel calmer, but you will be no use in a crisis.

The problem is that this ancient system isn't so useful in the modern world. There aren't many actual tigers around these days. Instead we face metaphorical tigers, such as deadlines, money worries, moving to a new house or getting to work on time.

These social threats trigger the same primal response, and while it makes perfect sense that you can't sleep during a tiger attack, it's much less helpful when faced with an angry boss or an exam in the morning.

THE EFFECTS OF STRESS

Although stress isn't a disease, staying in a constant state of emergency is quite bad for your health, and you need to manage it.

Stress affects your nervous system, redirecting energy from your body's "rest and digest" systems that keep you well and toward the "fight-or-flight" emergency systems that deal with the threat. After all, who cares about catching a cold when a tiger is eating you? Spend too long that way though, and it can cause long-term health issues, from coughs and colds to heart disease and organ damage.

Stress affects your mind too. In an effort to focus on the threat, you get tunnel vision and miss things around you. This makes sense – spotting a threat is more urgent than spotting an opportunity – but it makes it harder to think straight, learn new things, come up with ideas or solve complex problems.

Stress changes how you see risks and rewards. Stress is a state of action, a sign that you need to do something. When you're under

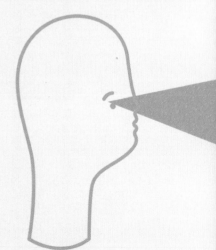

stress your mind will miss potential risks and focus only on rewards, making you more likely to act, but also more likely to make mistakes. When you're stressed, you are more likely to do stupid things and end up regretting things later.

MANAGING STRESS

It isn't possible to live completely without stress. If you care about things and want to get on in your career, take on challenges or improve your life, the chances are you will get stressed from time to time. If you like to work to the limit of your abilities, all it takes is one unexpected crisis and you can tip into stress. All you can do is manage the stress when it occurs, keep calm and minimize its impact.

Stress is your mind's emergency system.
It doesn't care what the emergency is though,
so you react to every threat as if it's a tiger attack.

STRESS: PHYSICAL SIGNS

- HEADACHES
- INSOMNIA
- DRY MOUTH
- EXHAUSTION
- POUNDING HEART

STRESS: PSYCHOLOGICAL SIGNS

- SHORT TEMPER
- HYPERACTIVITY
- RISK TAKING
- DIFFICULTY THINKING
- LOSS OF PERSPECTIVE

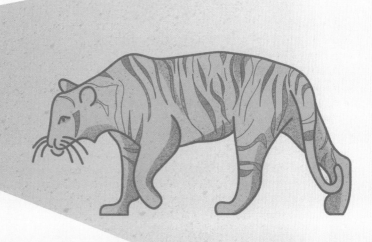

1. Know when you're stressed

Learning to spot the signs of stress (see page 39) can help you to deal with it quickly when it occurs. You won't have all of these symptoms, but if you spot one then you may notice others. If you start snapping at people or getting headaches, then check your decisions and watch your sleep patterns too.

2. Find the source

Stress is a sign that you feel overwhelmed, that you don't have the resources you need to deal with a situation. Unlike anxiety, which is a general fear of potential threats, stress always has a focus. If you are stressed, there is something in your life that is making you feel threatened, and you need to figure out what that is. Lots of things can make you stressed, but a few ingredients seem to trigger it:

- **SOMETHING YOU CARE ABOUT: Situations are only stressful if they matter to you, so it is often when you are most motivated and enthusiastic, or care most about other people or doing a good job, that you are vulnerable to stress.**
- **BEING WATCHED: Anything that threatens your status in the eyes of other people can be more stressful. In some studies, even someone standing in the corner of the room made people worse at complex tasks. Even making a cup of coffee can feel impossible if someone is standing behind you, criticizing your barista skills.**
- **LACK OF CONTROL: Stress is a feeling of powerlessness, that there is something that is beyond your ability to control. When the things that matter to you feel like they are slipping out of control, you will get stressed.**

3. Get perspective

Stress narrows your perspective, so when you're under stress you end up fixating on the problem and forgetting about the tools and resources you have to deal with it. You forget your skills, your friends, your experience, and end up clinging to the few resources you can see – making you even more stressed.

Breaking this vicious circle of lost perspective is fundamental to handling stress effectively. Remind yourself what you are good at, the people and assets you can call on to help you, and think about how you can use them to address the source of the problem. Reducing stress is a matter of deliberately shifting your focus from the threat itself to the tools you can use to deal with the threat.

You won't eliminate stress in one simple exercise, but by continuing to remind yourself of the things you're good at, and of the people who might be able to help you, you can reduce stress and turn pressures into challenges. You'll learn more about managing and building your resources in Chapter 8 (see page 130).

When you feel stressed, your focus narrows and you forget about the tools and resources that might help you. Consciously broadening your focus can remind you of your resources, and turn threats into challenges.

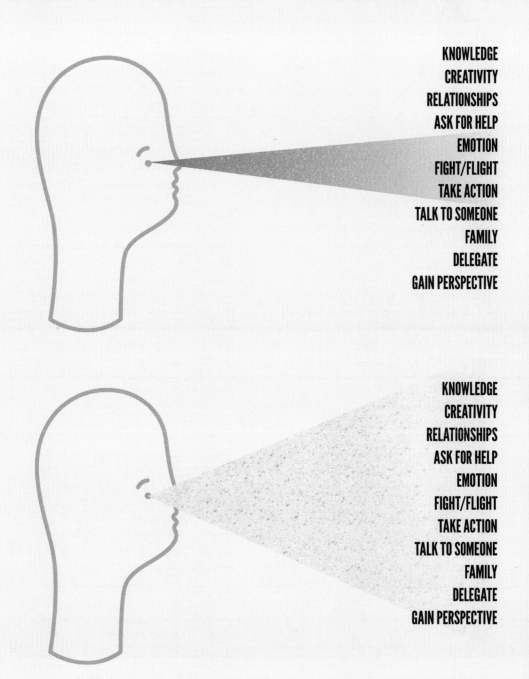

KNOWLEDGE
CREATIVITY
RELATIONSHIPS
ASK FOR HELP
EMOTION
FIGHT/FLIGHT
TAKE ACTION
TALK TO SOMEONE
FAMILY
DELEGATE
GAIN PERSPECTIVE

KNOWLEDGE
CREATIVITY
RELATIONSHIPS
ASK FOR HELP
EMOTION
FIGHT/FLIGHT
TAKE ACTION
TALK TO SOMEONE
FAMILY
DELEGATE
GAIN PERSPECTIVE

ANGER

Stress and anger are two sides of the same coin: when something is wrong, you can respond with fear (the urge to escape the problem) or anger (the urge to fight back). In fact, anger can be a response to fear, a way to calm anxiety or to push back against stress – the "fight" part of the fight-or-flight response.

Anger is one of the most destructive forces in the world. And yet, anger can be useful. It is a state of action, a drive to fix a problem. In controlled forms, it can help you identify what matters to you, indicate when your boundaries have been crossed and give you the energy to change things for the better.

The problem comes when anger takes over. Like stress, when you get angry you enter a heightened state, in which your emotions take over and you struggle to think clearly. Instead of responding accurately and appropriately, you may overreact or misunderstand what's happening, creating further problems. Like stress, anger is useful sometimes, but it needs to be managed.

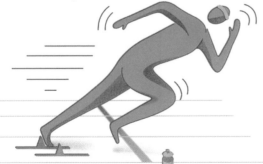

AVOIDING ANGER

You can't do much about the things that frustrate you in life, but you can manage yourself and your environment to reduce your chances of tipping into rage. Here are a few things that can make you less vulnerable to anger:

- **STAY FRESH:** Things get to you more when you're feeling unwell, your attention is spread thinly or your mental energy is low. At times like this it's hard to control your reactions and you are more likely to react badly. Something that drives you crazy one day can feel trivial the next, and the only difference might be a good night's sleep.

- **KEEP COOL:** You are more likely to get angry when you are already excited or worried. High-speed police chases, for example, are more likely to turn violent because of the fear and adrenaline of the chase. Keeping cool might even be a physical thing: you are more likely to react angrily when the weather is hot, because your body is already in a heightened state. Having an overheated mind isn't good for precision or reflection.

- **LET IT GO:** Sometimes things can make you angry because they remind you of something else that also made you angry. Instead of reacting proportionately to the event, you overreact, raging at things that aren't there. Whether it's stories from your past or something that happened this morning, try to let things go and approach each situation anew.

MANAGING ANGER

There is always something annoying, frustrating or downright maddening to draw your anger. So in addition to avoiding anger, you also need a plan for managing it when it strikes.

Anger is an instinctive response, the sprinter (see page 14) at its fastest and least focused. The thinker (see page 15) follows behind, trying to make sense of what's happening.

Managing anger is a matter of being aware of your anger and taking control of it before you do any damage. You need to use your cool thinker to rein in your overheating sprinter. Below are a few simple steps to get your anger back under control:

1. Accept your anger

You can't stop your first response – it happens without thinking – so the best thing you can do is acknowledge it, and don't try to bottle it up. You aren't accountable for how you feel, only the things you do, so give yourself permission to be angry.

2. Express your feelings safely

Ranting and raving isn't as cathartic as people think, but expressing your anger does seem to help people calm down. A 2010 Canadian study found people who expressed their anger constructively, by channelling it to something positive, suffered fewer health problems. Other studies suggest that expressing anger can be good for releasing energy and calming you down. Don't bottle it up. Just take care in how your expressions of anger affect other people.

3. Get clear on what's happening

When you feel angry, you are more likely to think of other things that make you angry,

creating a vicious circle. Try to interrupt this by thinking through what exactly is happening, and clear your mind of additional prompts for anger. The more able you are to get an accurate understanding of what is really making you angry right now, the more appropriate your response will be.

4. Get your thinker going

You don't need to let go of the feeling of anger, but you do need to engage your intellectual faculties. Counting to ten can help, but so can anything that engages your mind, such as doing mental arithmetic or remembering the actors in your favourite TV show. Try anything you can to get yourself thinking. Above all, try not to react right away. Take a breath, wait it out. Control your immediate reaction and give your second response time to reflect on the situation. Then if you still feel angry, respond appropriately.

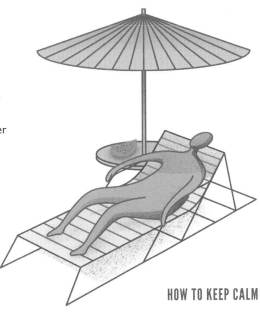

DON'T FEAR YOUR ANGER

Your emotions are signals telling you what you need, so explore why you're angry and use that information to help you respond better. Is it something that's happened just now, or are you angry about an accumulation of things? What would be a proportionate response? And how do other people see the situation?

Learn what happens in your mind when you get angry. What is your first response when you get angry? What goes through your mind, and what do you want to do? And what about your second response? What do you end up thinking later on, once you've had a bit of time to calm down and consider things properly?

Remember, you aren't accountable for what goes through your mind, only for what you do as a result.

DAMAGE LIMITATION

Of course, you can't control your anger all the time. Sometimes you will simply be too angry to think clearly or control your behaviour.

In these situations the best thing you can do is to limit the damage to yourself and others. Take yourself out of the situation, and then have the humility to apologize afterward if you have overreacted. Remember, we all get angry, and we all react; no one expects you to be an emotionless robot. What matters is having the wisdom to notice when you've gone too far, and the courage to say sorry.

Above all, stay safe. Anger can lead to violence, and other extreme responses that feel right at the time, but are appalling in the cold light of day. Don't take your anger out on other people, and don't be tempted to seek revenge on those who hurt you. You will get things wrong, make a mistake and end up regretting it.

There will always be annoying things in life, and you will get angry. Other people being rude or careless, problems at work, road rage and people letting you down – all these things and more can press your buttons. Think about what makes you angry, and ask yourself why. If there are principles to defend, or boundaries to maintain, then a little anger can be healthy. As for the rest, though, try to let it go.

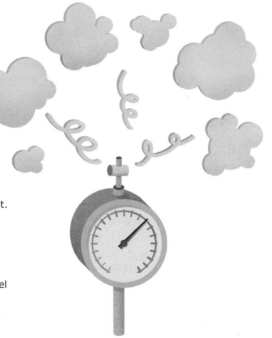

MOODS

We use the word "mood" a lot – "He's in a mood", "I'm in a good mood" and so on – but we hardly ever consider what it means. Moods are subtly different from emotions, like fear and anger, and require a slightly different approach.

Moods are background feelings, rather like an emotional body temperature. In fact, we even use the word in the same way. You always have some sort of mood, just like you always have a body temperature. It's only when there's something unusual about it that you say you're in a mood, or have a temperature.

Emotions come and go, but moods are more persistent and can hang around for hours or even days. They affect your emotions, and vice versa. Both can give you useful insights into how the events in your life are affecting you.

The influential mood researchers William Morris and Randy Larsen saw moods and emotions as two different kinds of information. Emotions give you information about how you feel about the events in your life; moods give you information about your inner state and what you have taken on from events in your life.

UNDERSTANDING YOUR MOODS

Managing your moods can help you to manage the impact the world has on your mind. Good habits of mood management can help you shake off things that have worried you, and avoid intense emotional reactions.

Moods are linked to your autonomic nervous system, the driver of responses such as stress and excitement. Although we talk about "good" and "bad" moods, we can actually measure mood in two dimensions: comfort and energy. You can feel good, but tired; and you can feel bad, but full of energy. These two drivers, energy and comfort, drive your behaviour and link mind and body together.

Tuning into your mood is tricky, but it is very useful. Think about how much energy you have right now. Do you feel full of energy or a bit flat? How comfortable do you feel? Do you feel at ease, free from troubles, or are things playing on your mind and making you worried or annoyed? Knowing your moods is a powerful tool for self-management. If you know, on a day-to-day basis, how energized and relaxed you are feeling, you will be more aware of how your emotional state is affecting your mind, and your behaviour.

There are many different factors that affect your moods:

- **YOUR PERSONALITY:** Sensitive people (see page 22) are often more affected by negative events. Agreeable people (see page 26) may be more likely to take on moods from around them. Everyone has different natural set points for their moods, so it can be very personal.
- **BODY CHEMISTRY:** Hormones can make you feel tense or tired, wake you up or calm you down. Since moods are quite physical, they are affected by what you eat and drink too, especially mood-altering substances such as caffeine, sugar and alcohol.
- **OTHER PEOPLE:** We are sensitive to other people's moods and emotions. If someone

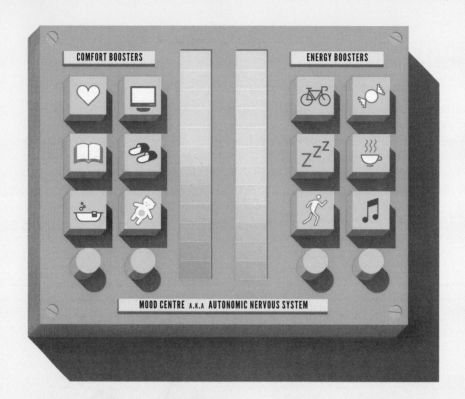

COMFORT BOOSTERS

ENERGY BOOSTERS

MOOD CENTRE A.K.A AUTONOMIC NERVOUS SYSTEM

near you is tired, you will feel tired too; if people are nervous, you can take on their nervousness. Moods seem to be sociable.

● EVENTS AND EMOTIONS: The pressures you are under and the things on your mind can build up, subtly affecting how you feel in the long term.

MOOD MANAGEMENT

Moods have a natural rhythm, and it is not always possible to control your inner state. Obsessing about your moods can be unhealthy: you don't need to be over-vigilant. Just try to tune into your mind and body and notice how you're feeling, and build a routine to keep yourself feeling good.

Managing your moods proactively isn't all that easy. They are longer lasting than emotions, harder to identify and less connected to external events, so you can't manage them consciously like you can stress or anger.

Research on mood regulation argues that we all manage our moods through our daily actions, though often without even realizing it. You do things to make yourself feel comfortable, soothing your mind and relaxing your body; and you do things to raise your energy and recharge your mind.

Psychologist Robert Thayer, in his book *Calm Energy*, suggests that a lot of our day-to-day actions are about mood management, and particularly avoiding discomfort.

Many of the things we do habitually are designed to avoid uncomfortable moods, including lots of compulsive behaviours. We drink coffee and eat sugary foods to give us energy, and drink wine and smoke cigarettes to calm ourselves down. The list of things people say they do to manage their moods reads like a list of every public health problem imaginable. Every addiction, from sugar fixes to smoking, can be a form of mood management.

ADAPT YOUR DAILY ROUTINE

Think about what you do to manage your moods. What do you do in the morning to wake yourself up? What do you do when you hit an afternoon lull? What about when you feel nervous and need to relax?

Some people prefer gentle activities such as music and gardening, while others prefer more energetic pursuits such as dancing and sports. The things you do to manage your moods are personal and vary with culture, way of life, interests and personality.

The most important thing is to identify what works for you. We generally do whatever feels easiest and most comfortable, so your self-management behaviours need to fit in with your way of life. Find your own relaxing "breathers" and energizing "restorers", and build them into your daily routine, to maintain your emotional wellbeing and keep yourself focused and productive.

Managing your moods can help you get ahead of your emotions and turn calm energy into a habit. Stay on top of your moods, and you will be less likely to feel angry or stressed, overreact to situations, and end up ruled by your emotions.

MONITOR YOUR MOODS

Moods and emotions are important though, and they should not be suppressed or "fixed". We may need to put these messages aside to get things done, but we ignore them at our peril. Any emotion can be healthy and useful in the right context, and sometimes the most appropriate response is to feel tense or tired.

Listen to your mind and notice what it needs to be calm and effective, but don't worry too much about trying to stay in one particular mood all the time. The key is to understand and process your moods effectively, to manage your activities and routine accordingly, and not to get stuck for too long in unhelpful feelings.

Use your moods to monitor how you are feeling, and then let them go when they are no longer useful to you. As Randy Larsen put it, you need to learn how to hang up the phone, after getting the message.

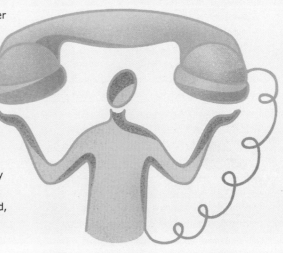

SELF-REGULATION

The deliberate and habitual ways in which we manage our emotions through our actions is known in psychology as "self-regulation". Self-regulation is not a tool for emergencies, but a good habit to develop in life. Whether you want to feel better, get more done or have better relationships, self-regulation can help you get some influence over how you feel, rather than being a slave to your emotions.

SURFACE ACTING AND DEEP ACTING

The simplest way to manage your emotions is to fake it. This is sometimes called surface acting: pretending to feel one thing when you actually feel something else. We can become surprisingly good at doing this, putting on a brave face, smiling at a bad joke or looking serious in a meeting. The trouble is, surface acting is tiring and takes conscious effort, a kind of emotional labour that can drain you of mental energy. You can do it for a while, but eventually you end up exhausted.

A better method is deep acting, shifting your emotional state through your thoughts and actions. Rather than pretending to be sad at a funeral, tune into the sadness around you and feel sad with everyone else. Managing your emotions in this way is a far more efficient and effective way to manage how you feel.

EMOTIONAL INTELLIGENCE

There is no quick fix for managing your emotions: different strategies work for different feelings. Every situation is different

and no one can tell you exactly what will work best in any given situation. Self-regulation must be learned.

A common term for this capacity to spot and manage emotions is emotional intelligence. It is important for maintaining wellbeing, having good relationships and generally being successful in life and work. It's particularly useful in social settings, when you need to watch what you say or mind your reactions. Learning when and how to express your emotions, both good and bad, is an important aspect of social and emotional intelligence.

Emotions are mainly the domain of the sprinter (see page 14), the fast, instinctive part of your mind. Whenever something significant happens, you will have a feeling about it. It might not be intense or noticeable, but it will be there: an instinct to approach things you like, avoid things you don't, fight things that scare you, and so on. You can't control your emotions. You can't take the credit for how you feel, so you don't get the blame either.

COGNITIVE BEHAVIOURAL THERAPY

One of the big breakthroughs in emotional self-management came in the 1960s in the work of the psychiatrist Aaron Beck. Frustrated with the focus in traditional psychotherapy on childhood trauma and deep-rooted problems, Beck developed a therapy that focused instead on coping strategies and dealing with difficult emotions and behaviours. The result was Cognitive Behavioural Therapy (CBT).

The underlying principle of CBT is that your thoughts and actions affect your feelings. Your feelings, in turn, affect your thoughts and behaviour, creating unhelpful patterns and feedback loops – what Beck termed the cognitive triangle. You can't control your feelings, but you can control the way you think, and how you respond. Manage your thoughts and behaviour, and the feelings will follow.

The trick with self-regulation is to accept your first response, and not add to it with a second response. Clear your mind of negative thought patterns and you will have a clearer understanding of how things are making you feel. This isn't about becoming numb or ignoring your feelings: it's about clearing your mind of additional noise, so you can figure out how the situation is really making you feel.

A key part of this is "cognitive distancing", noticing your thoughts but not being lost in them. It is the difference between thinking "This is stupid" and "I am having the thought that this is stupid". Cognitive distancing allows you to accept and experience your feelings, but still choose whether to act on them or not.

Rather than being separate systems, thoughts and feelings are deeply related, and both affect your behaviour – just as your behaviour can change how you think and feel too.

THOUGHTS

FEELINGS

BEHAVIOUR

LIVING IN THE NOW

Anger, fear and discomfort are in many ways different responses to the same underlying problem: wishing the world was other than how it is. Whether we mean to or not, we compare the world to how it used to be, or what we want it to be like, and when the world doesn't match our expectations, we feel upset.

This is a problem that has preoccupied many thinkers over the years. Stoic philosophers, Christian ascetics, Muslim contemplatives and Chinese sages have all wrestled with it, but the person whose work has left the deepest mark is that of Gautama Siddhartha, the Buddha.

Buddha developed his ideas in and around ancient India in the fifth century BCE, but his influence stretches far beyond that culture. There are many interpretations of Buddha's work, but at a very basic level he taught that the reason we suffer is because we get attached to how we wish the world was, and neglect how it is. These attachments cause us discomfort, but by meditating on present experiences, we can let go of our desires and live in the moment, free from fear, sadness or anger.

MINDFULNESS

Modern pioneers in the field of meditation such as John Kabat-Zinn, Sharon Salzberg and Joseph Goldstein have taken the ancient wisdom of Buddhism and other contemplative traditions and fashioned it into modern, secular programmes. One of the best techniques for handling stress, anger and anxiety is to take your attention off the past or the future, and focus it on the present moment. This non-judgmental awareness of the present moment is called "mindfulness".

The core of mindfulness is training your attention, deliberately putting your focus on your breath, your body, the world around you or other things in your experience. It isn't about emptying your mind, or tuning things out; in fact it is precisely the opposite. We spend so much of our time sleepwalking through life, preoccupied with things we're worried about, but if we really pay attention to all the many things in the world around us, there isn't room for worry as well. Even making a cup of tea is an intense process, full of smells, tastes, feelings and so on.

Think of mindfulness as a way to get real, to see the world as it is

If you put the hours in, the benefits of regular mindfulness meditation are extensive. A 2013 study concluded that mindfulness-based therapy is especially effective for reducing anxiety, depression and stress. The University of Utah found mindfulness could help people control their emotions and sleep better.

Research by professor of psychology and psychiatry Richard Davidson even found that people showed changes in their brain patterns after just eight weeks of mindfulness-based stress reduction, with less activation in areas associated with stress, anxiety and depression, and more in areas associated with feeling calm and happy.

There are many more ways to be present in the moment than meditation though, and there is still some debate about whether meditative practice actually makes people more mindful in daily life. Mindfulness doesn't work for everyone: some people find it makes them more upset, or just has no effect.

Mindfulness is not a command to accept everything the world throws at you either. Sometimes the right thing to do is to get angry, or make plans to avoid disaster. Appreciating the world doesn't prevent you from changing it.

Instead, it may be better to think of mindfulness as a way to get real, to see the world as it is. You may still find things you don't like or want to change, but at least they are real things. There's quite enough to be worried or angry about in the real world without imagining new problems in your head too.

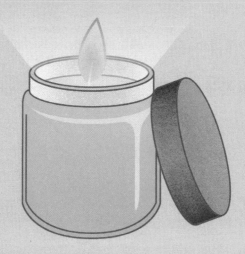

A QUIET LIFE?

At the heart of all this lies a curious lesson about human nature. We want two things from life: excitement and comfort.

We have one emotional system for feeling excited, driven by natural stimulants such as dopamine, and another that brings us comfort, driven by the calming influence of serotonin. The neuroeconomist Baba Shiv argues that these twin drivers, excitement and comfort, define our choices and shape our lives.

The best moments come when we find something that gives us both, such as a new relationship or a fun rollercoaster. Most of the time, though, we must choose. Sometimes we want excitement, to avoid boredom and apathy. Other times we want comfort, to avoid stress, anxiety and anger. As Keith Johnstone, one of the pioneers of improvised theatre, put it, there is a world of yes and a world of no. One leads to adventure, the other leads to safety.

Some of us prefer a quiet life, avoiding risks in return for feeling calm and free from worry. Others put up with being stressed and anxious because it's more fun than being bored. But life is short, and it can be better to be uncomfortable and experience life, than live in a bubble and miss the opportunities around you.

Excitement and comfort: two drivers that shape our experiences. Do you prefer pressure to boredom? Rest over adventure? What sort of life do you want?

EXCITEMENT

PRESSURE

ADVENTURE

COMFORT

BOREDOM

REST

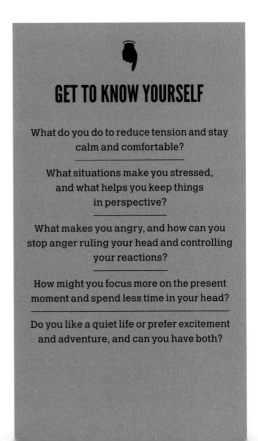

GET TO KNOW YOURSELF

What do you do to reduce tension and stay calm and comfortable?

What situations make you stressed, and what helps you keep things in perspective?

What makes you angry, and how can you stop anger ruling your head and controlling your reactions?

How might you focus more on the present moment and spend less time in your head?

Do you like a quiet life or prefer excitement and adventure, and can you have both?

WHAT WORKS FOR YOU?

Find a place to be silent and sit there for a while.

Slow down.

Look up at the night sky.

Body scan my emotions.

Write a daily journal (anything that comes up; don't censor).

HOW TO BE HAPPY

THE PURSUIT OF HAPPINESS

Have you ever wondered why silver medallists look so unhappy? In 1994, the psychologists Victoria Medvec, Scott Madey and Thomas Gilovich analysed the facial expressions of Olympic medal winners on the podium. Gold and bronze medallists looked happy, but silver medallists tended to look less pleased. Coming in second was worse than coming in third.

The reason, they said, lay in counterfactuals. Silver medallists are sad not to win gold, while bronze medallists are glad not to be fourth. This is the challenge of happiness: we don't compare our lives to some abstract gold standard, but to how we imagine our lives should be.

GAINS AND LOSSES

In the 1970s and 1980s, the psychologists Amos Tversky and Daniel Kahneman, in their Nobel prize-winning work on prospect theory, proposed that satisfaction with our choices comes not from how much we have, but from our gains and losses. Kahneman has said judgment works rather like vision: we notice movements and pay less attention to maintained states. So when it comes to happiness, we focus on changes and ignore things that stay the same.

A 2016 McKinsey Global Institute survey of six thousand people in France, Britain and America found this is even true of money. Our happiness depends less on what we have, and more on whether we feel we are making progress, doing better than in the past. It is not poverty by itself that causes unhappiness, but its by-product, worrying about not having enough money. Having more money can alleviate poverty, but it won't necessarily stop you from worrying about becoming poor.

Happiness is not a fixed point, but a matter of comparison

In the 1970s, the psychologists Philip Brickman and Donald Campbell found that even major life events don't seem to affect our long-term happiness. Winning the lottery makes you happy for a while, and a serious accident can make you unhappy. But within a couple of years you will have got used to your gains or losses and feel the same as before. Your big win won't be as exciting once you are used to having more money, and that serious accident will feel less traumatic when you have adapted to the life that follows. Brickman and Campbell called this effect the hedonic treadmill, our tendency to adjust to things and keep moving.

A MATTER OF PERSPECTIVE

It is encouraging to know we are resilient to adversity. We are actually much better than we think at recovering from bad experiences. The trouble is, we seem to be resilient to happiness too. If you believe your life will be better with that amazing new house, great job or more cash in the bank, you may end up being disappointed. Happiness is not a fixed point, but a matter of comparison – to other people, to your expectations, to the past.

And yet, happiness remains as popular a goal as ever. Products are sold by promising it; we make life choices in the hope of attaining it; whole countries are dedicated to the pursuit of it. Happiness is something we all want, for ourselves and for the people we love.

So if happiness is just a matter of perspective, why aren't we happier? Of course, lack of money, safety, food, shelter and other basic ingredients of life matter, but, in the developed world at least, we have more comforts than ever before, and yet happiness is no higher than it was. So how are we managing to live so well and yet be so unhappy? What can we do to get the happiness we seek? And what is happiness anyway?

DEFINING HAPPINESS

Happiness is a difficult concept to pin down. For some people it means to feel cheerful and upbeat, to enjoy the day and have a positive outlook. Other people think about happiness in more profound terms, speaking of deep satisfaction and a meaningful life. Somewhere amid these different ideas is a unifying concept of flourishing, living well and enjoying experiences. Psychologists often refer to this collection of ideas as "subjective wellbeing", a sense that you are enjoying your life each day.

Why would it be worse to come second than third? Because happiness is less about what you have, and more about your expectations.

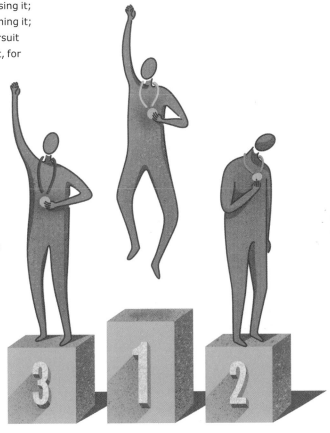

ENJOY YOUR MIND

mindapples

A FORMULA FOR HAPPINESS?

Your wellbeing and happiness levels seem to come from a combination of factors.

Genetics do matter, of course. If you are a naturally extroverted person (see page 20), and particularly if you are lower in sensitivity to negative emotions (see page 22), you can find yourself being happy more often. There isn't an exact science to how your brain chemistry affects your happiness (it may be different for different areas of your life), but it does seem that we start from slightly different set points in our quest for wellbeing. We can all be happy, but some of us have to work a little harder than others.

Upbringing seems to have an effect too, but not perhaps as much as we used to think. The old view of psychology, that who we are as adults is shaped by our experiences in childhood, seems to be over-simplistic. It helps to have a good family and not to have struggled too much earlier in life, but trauma and serious problems, although they may still affect you, won't define you.

The rest of your happiness is down to your daily actions, life choices and other things you do. You can't change everything about your happiness, but a large proportion of how you feel day-to-day is in your hands.

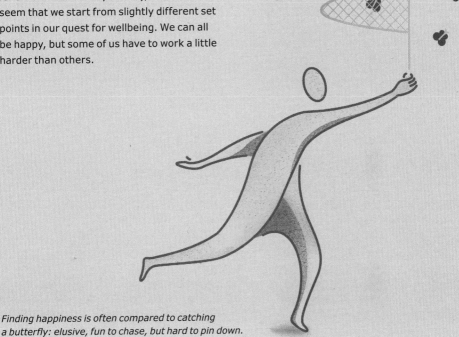

Finding happiness is often compared to catching a butterfly: elusive, fun to chase, but hard to pin down.

HAPPY HABITS

Happiness is personal and there isn't a simple recipe you can follow to make you happier. However, there are a few activities that seem to boost happiness and wellbeing.

SMILE

Smiling is a signal of feeling good, so seeing people smile can cheer you up. What's stranger though, is that smiling seems to cheer up the person smiling too: if you force yourself to smile then eventually your mood catches up.

GO OUTSIDE

Natural light is good for boosting your mood, producing vitamin D and getting your mind going. People who go without natural daylight may end up feeling flat, lacking in energy and even a bit depressed. You don't need blazing sunshine: just go outside and look around.

SEE YOUR FAMILY AND FRIENDS

Other people are crucial for your happiness. Spending time with people you love and trust is one of the best mood boosters there is.

PLAY

Happiness isn't a serious business. There are lots of things that can make you feel happier, but all of them work better if you enjoy them. Make time for fun, and happiness will follow.

PLAN THINGS YOU ENJOY

Having fun is great, but so too is planning it. A 2010 study found that planning a holiday was actually more fun than going on holiday. Imagining wonderful things may be just as good as them happening in real life – but try not to lose yourself completely in fantasy.

SHARE THE JOY

A 2012 study found that happy memories have a much stronger effect on your mood if you share them with other people. Sharing good experiences doubles the fun, and you'll be more likely to remember them later too.

HELP PEOPLE

Happiness isn't a selfish exercise. Volunteering, being useful to others and helping people out all seem to help boost mood and wellbeing. Even small gestures can work. Want to be happy? Make someone else happy.

BE GRATEFUL

Research by Robert Emmons, a psychologist at the University of California, and many others, has found huge benefits to being grateful. Grateful people tend to have stronger relationships, be less materialistic and be

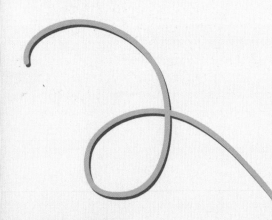

more generous. You don't necessarily have to tell other people: even making a list of the things you're grateful for each day seems to be good for building happiness and positivity.

KEEP BUSY
We may enjoy doing nothing, but generally we seem to be happier when we're busy, particularly doing something that uses our skills and energy. This may explain why people take a while to adjust to retirement, and also why unemployment is terrible for happiness.

HAVE A GOOD CRY
Crying can be a great way to cheer yourself up. A study published in 2011 found that intense crying put people in a positive mood, and that crying in the company of another person was even better.

HUG A TEDDY
If crying doesn't work, try hugging a teddy bear. According to a 2011 experiment, it can reduce feelings of loneliness and isolation, and might even make you like people again.

WILL CHANGING YOUR LIFE MAKE YOU HAPPIER?

We are surprisingly bad at predicting what will make us happy. In a 1998 study, the psychologists David Schkade and Daniel Kahneman asked people in Ohio and California whether they thought people who lived in Ohio or California were happier. Both groups said people living in California were happier – but in fact, both were equally happy. You might think moving to the coast will transform your life, but it could be a lot of effort for nothing.

There is perhaps a good reason for this: if small life changes made you happier, then they could make you miserable too. We are naturally resilient, to good things and bad. One study conducted by the behavioural geneticist David Lykken in 1996 even concluded that trying to be happier is as futile as trying to be taller.

Studies by the positive psychologists Sonja Lyubomirsky and Kennon Sheldon suggest that changing your life circumstances might not be the best way to increase happiness. If you are already moderately comfortable, then what really affects your happiness are your habits, the things you do and the way you think.

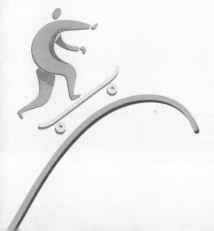

CHEER UP!

One of the most annoying questions ever asked is "Are you a glass-half-full or a glass-half-empty person?" This question is often asked by people who are cheerful all the time, and who are afraid of empty glasses. There is a place for positive thinking: thinking positively can counteract biases in your thinking and stop you getting lost in problems. Just don't take it too far.

THE POWER OF POSITIVE THINKING

While traditional psychology has focused on illness and problems, positive psychology works by building people's strengths rather than fixing weaknesses. The influential positive psychologist Martin Seligman and colleagues have even proposed forms of positive therapy, and have devised programmes to help people be the best version of themselves.

Optimistic thinking can improve your life

Optimistic thinking can improve your life, rather than the other way around. Thinking positively seems to help us notice our successes and learn to repeat them, and gives us the headspace to learn new things and build our resources.

Seligman has proposed the idea of learned helplessness – the theory that we can become conditioned to feeling trapped, useless and unable to help ourselves. How far these habits are learned, and how much they can be changed, is unclear, but positive thinking certainly seems to help break people out of these negative spirals.

HOW TO BECOME MORE POSITIVE

Your mind can run away with you, thinking more negatively until it becomes a habit. To counteract this, here are some ways to build new habits of positive thinking:

1. Focus on what you can control
What are your strengths, and what changes can you make to your life? You can't control everything, but there's usually something you can do differently.

2. Think about what you like about your life
This can be hard when you feel miserable. Think about the people in your life, the activities you enjoy, the things you've achieved. Things may not be perfect, but they probably aren't perfectly awful either.

3. Appreciate the happy people in your life
Think about the people who cheer you up, and spend more time with them. Sometimes just being around people who are happy can rub off on you, reminding you of good things and building optimistic thinking.

4. Try doing things that are enjoyable and useful
If you don't feel happy, try making someone else feel happy. Find enjoyable things to do

that will also make you feel useful to people. Very often, the key to happiness isn't selfish pleasure: it is altruism.

5. Focus on what you have, not what you don't have

If you don't have much money, think about what other assets you do have, such as skills and relationships. It doesn't mean you don't need the other things, but it can help to remind you of what you've got.

DON'T BE AFRAID OF NEGATIVITY

Positive thinking isn't everything though. Feeling flat or sad is quite healthy, and optimism doesn't have to mean being unrealistic. So what if the glass is half empty? What's so bad about empty glasses anyway? Empty glasses are useful: there are lots of things you can do with all that space.

In fact, resisting bad moods could make them worse. In a 2014 study, researchers interviewed 365 people about their attitudes to their emotions, and then monitored their moods for three weeks. All the participants had their ups and downs, but the people who had negative attitudes toward their bad moods had more trouble and health problems than those who accepted their bad moods. In other words, try to be positive, but be positive about negativity too.

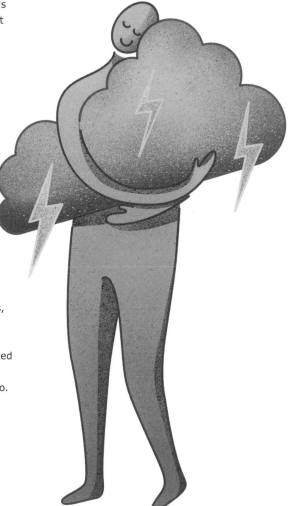

THE JOY OF SADNESS

Positive thinking has grown in popularity lately, but it isn't for everyone. The risk with happiness is that it can feel like telling people to cheer up rather than improving their lives.

In her 2010 book *Bright-sided: How Positive Thinking Is Undermining America*, Barbara Ehrenreich criticizes the self-help movement for making people delusional and prone to blaming others unfairly for their problems.

Indeed, there may be a moral imperative to being unhappy. If you see terrible things happening in the world, it isn't always good to shrug them off. Criticism and dissent are important tools for making positive change.

There's some evidence that positive thinking can make people feel worse too. A 2010 study found that some self-help books can make sensitive people (see page 22) feel more insecure, and a 2009 study found self-help mantras can be bad for people with low self-esteem. Visualizing future successes can reduce your motivation too, because it gives you a fantasy of success and takes away your desire to make your goals a reality.

The other risk with positive thinking is that it might make us intolerant of negative emotions. Happiness campaigns and self-help books, if done badly, can create a pressure to be happy. Keep thinking positively or you will be miserable – and if you are, it's your fault for not believing hard enough.

BEING SAD CAN BE GOOD FOR YOU

Negative emotions are a part of a healthy mind. In fact, if you are never sad, there's probably something wrong with you. Emotions such as happiness and sadness are not simply there to be enjoyed or avoided: they give you valuable information about how you feel about the events in your life, and they can focus your attention on what matters.

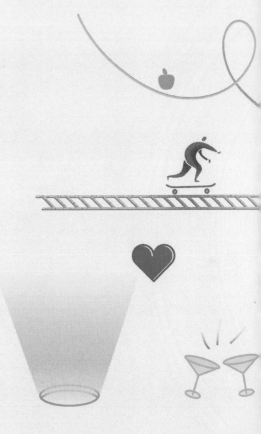

The broaden-and-build theory, developed by the psychologist Barbara Fredrickson, argues that positive emotions signal that we are safe and able to explore. They can help us learn new things, think creatively, make connections and build new relationships. Negative emotions do the opposite: they signal that something is wrong and focus your mind on problems. This can be just as useful, even if it is less pleasant.

In our collective pursuit of happiness, we often forget the benefits of feeling sad. Here are just a few reasons *not* to be cheerful:

1. Bad moods can motivate you

A 2011 study found that the most engaged people at work were those who started the day in a bad mood, and then took action to fix things. People who just felt happy saw less reason to act.

2. Sad people are more persuasive

When people are upset they get better at explaining issues to other people, capturing our attention, producing better arguments and convincing us of the need to change.

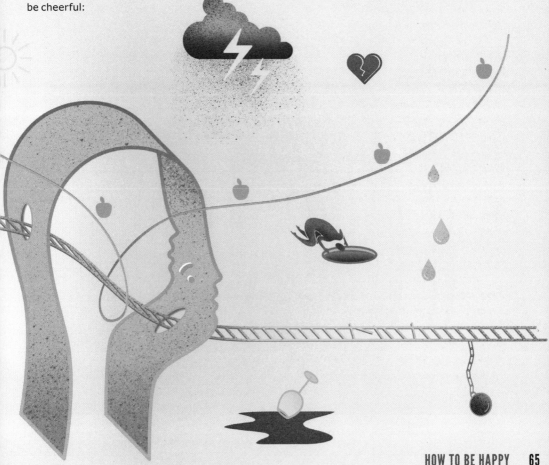

3. Sadness gives us empathy

A 2005 Canadian study found depressed people were better at noticing emotions in those around them. It's easier to support someone if you know what they're going through.

4. Sadness makes people thoughtful

A 2013 study found that people did better at analytic thinking when asked to do so by someone feeling sad, and more creative thinking when asked by someone happy.

5. Feeling bad can make you less gullible

Many studies have connected negative moods to scepticism and being less swayed by false information. When we feel bad we remember things better, ask more questions and spot lies. Rather than moaning, negative people may actually be seeing things more clearly.

NOTICE THE GOOD AS WELL AS THE BAD

The thing to be fought is not sadness, but bias. Negativity bias is your tendency to recall bad memories more easily than good memories. It is your mind's helpful instinct to keep you safe and fix problems, but it can lead to you missing the good stuff and thinking the world is more unpleasant or hostile than it really is.

In these situations, it can be helpful to correct your distortion by forcing yourself to think positively. This is one of the hardest (and the most irritating) things to have to do, but it can help you see the world more clearly and make better decisions.

Too much focus on happiness, though, without acknowledging the value of sadness, can be risky. There are many situations in which it is good to be sad, such as when you attend a funeral, for example (for more on sadness see pages 134–5).

Our desire to be happy shouldn't obscure the value of critical thought, or the need to promote mental health in the wider sense. The opposite of depression isn't happiness; it is balance. There's much more to leading a good life than just being cheerful.

Don't feel pressured to put on a brave face. Instead, think about how you can use your feelings constructively, and support people around you.

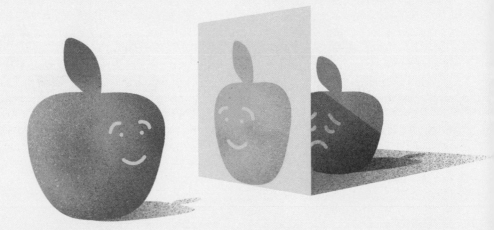

THE GOOD LIFE

The pursuit of happiness, then, is a complex and elusive business.

On one level, happiness is about feeling good and finding joy in the moment. The Ancient Greek philosopher Epicurus argued the ultimate goal of life is pleasure – to enjoy the experience of being alive – and there is certainly something to this. Although his ideas have been caricatured as meaning a life of greed and indulgence, Epicurus himself lived modestly, savouring the simple pleasures, advocating friendship and gratitude, and appreciating what he had. If he were alive today, there's a good chance Epicurus would be a positive psychologist.

Happiness isn't all about pleasure though. Plato, another Ancient Greek philosopher, said that constantly seeking pleasure is like being a leaky jug, always needing to be filled. This pursuit of happiness in the moment can, ironically, leave us feeling unhappy. In her book *The Ethics of Ambiguity*, the French philosopher Simone de Beauvoir cautioned against seeking shallow excitement and experiences without taking a moral stance or fighting for something important.

A MEANINGFUL LIFE

In his famous 1946 book *Man's Search for Meaning*, the Jewish psychiatrist and Holocaust survivor Viktor Frankl argues that what really matters in life is not pleasure, but meaning. If we have meaning in our lives, we can bear suffering in the present. Living pleasantly is less important than knowing why we are alive.

MAXIMIZERS AND SATISFICERS

The psychologist Barry Schwartz says that the reason we are often unhappy is because we have too much choice. There is always something else to try, a path not taken, or someone else who looks happier than you.

Some people seek to maximize their happiness by seeking out better and better choices and are always looking for the next improvement. Other people, argues Schwartz, just seek satisfaction. They decide what they want and seek it out – and once they have found it, they stop looking and enjoy what they have.

"Maximizers" are always finding new things to make them happy, but it is the "satisficers" who actually feel satisfied with their lives. Your happiness is less controlled by what you have, than by how content you are with what you have.

In 2013, research led by the social psychologist Roy Baumeister found that pleasure and meaning didn't always go hand in hand. It found that people who rated their lives as more meaningful also experienced more stress and worry. Many of us sacrifice short-term pleasures in order to achieve something important. Most parents say they would put up with personal unhappiness in order to make their children happier.

So what's going on here? Should you seek a life of pleasure, or a life of meaning?

Is happiness about enjoying life now,
or suffering for something that matters?

GOOD EXPERIENCES OR GOOD MEMORIES?
The psychologist Daniel Kahneman has a
theory to explain this. In his later work he has
come to believe that the way we've pursued and
studied happiness in the past is wrong, because
there are actually two kinds of happiness.
Your "experiencing self" wants pleasure in
the moment, to enjoy life now; while your
"remembering self" wants to look back and feel
satisfaction, a sense of having had a good life.
You think you want good experiences, he says,
but you actually want good memories.

Most of life is made up of routine experiences
that slip by unnoticed. Some we enjoy, and
some we don't, but both are quickly forgotten.
The events that stick in the mind tend to be the
extremes, the moments of great achievement
or hopeless despair. In a 2006 study of hospital
procedures, people's rating of how painful
a procedure was didn't seem to be based on
how they'd felt during it, but on whether the
pain was bad at the end. The experience was
lost; the memory is what mattered.

This may explain some of the riddles of
happiness research. Having more money might
give you a greater sense of satisfaction, but it
doesn't make you happier day-to-day. Pleasure
might be good in the moment, but it's not much
use when you're looking back over what you've
accomplished in your life. Good experiences
matter, and so do good memories; but to be
truly happy, you need both.

FOCUS ON WHAT MATTERS TO YOU
With so many factors at play, from momentary
pleasures to meaningful achievements,
happiness can feel like an impossible dream.
So perhaps the final thing to know in this quest
for happiness is that there is no such thing as
being perfectly happy. Life isn't about seeking
perfection: it is about figuring out what matters
to you, and learning to enjoy it.

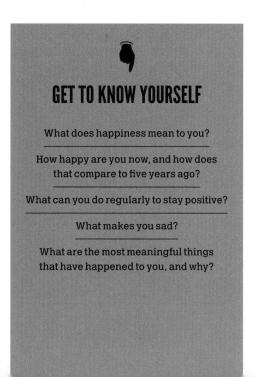

GET TO KNOW YOURSELF

What does happiness mean to you?

How happy are you now, and how does
that compare to five years ago?

What can you do regularly to stay positive?

What makes you sad?

What are the most meaningful things
that have happened to you, and why?

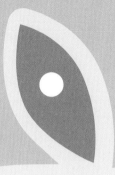

WHAT WORKS FOR YOU?

At the end of every day, think of
three good things that happened.

Wear bright colours.

Keep a gratitude diary
(write one thing each night).

Sing and dance.

Eat cake and don't care.

HOW TO HAVE A HEALTHY MIND

MIND YOUR HEAD

What's the first word that comes into your mind when you hear the term "mental health"? If you're like most people, you probably think about stress, depression and other health problems. For many people, mental health is even associated with madness, losing control and being afraid.

Now, what's the first word that springs to your mind when you hear the term "physical health"? The chances are you thought about getting fit, eating well and feeling in shape. Being physically healthy is actually quite sexy. Mental health, not so much.

These attitudes don't come out of nowhere. We are bombarded with messages about taking care of our bodies. We still learn about cancer, heart problems, the dangers of smoking and other health risks, but all this comes with a backdrop of positive imagery of keeping fit, feeling good and looking great.

Mental health doesn't get the same kind of press. It's certainly in the news more these days, but the culture remains fixed on problems, about how we need to talk about stress, depression and suicide, and the discrimination faced by people with mental health issues. These are all vitally important issues, just like cancer or heart disease, but when it comes to the health of our minds, we're still missing the positive side, the practical things we can do, and the positive images to inspire us.

HEALTHY MIND, HEALTHY BODY

Having a healthy mind should be as important to us as getting fit or eating well. In fact, having a healthy mind is essential for being physically healthy. Many of the things we do that are bad for our bodies – eating sugary and fatty foods, smoking, drinking, self-medicating, not exercising – stem from how we feel emotionally. We generally know what's good for our health: the great mystery is how hard we find it to put this knowledge into practice.

The mind can make the body sick too. Stress and depression can cause serious physical health issues such as heart attacks and back problems, and mental wellbeing has been linked to a whole range of physical health benefits such as better immune response, fewer coughs and colds, coping better with pain, better heart health, fighting serious illnesses and generally living a longer and happier life.

This isn't a book about how to be physically healthy though. Instead, we'll focus on this missing ingredient in health promotion: the psychological aspects of a healthy way of life.

Most people say their mental health is as important as their physical health – but how much do we really do to keep our minds in shape?

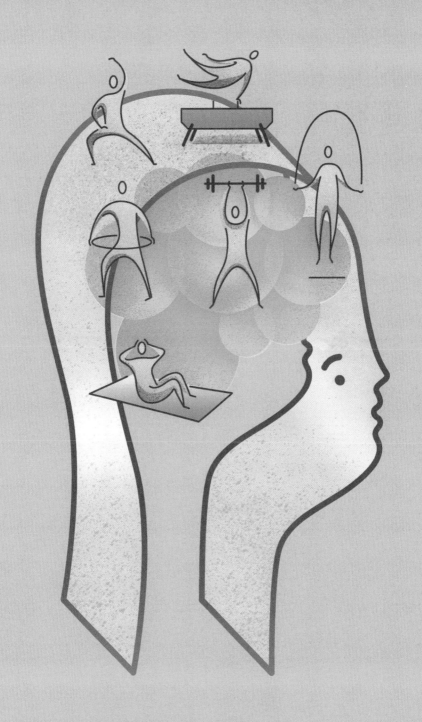

LOOKING AFTER YOUR MIND

Unlike physical health, we are taught very little about how to stay mentally healthy. But there are actually lots of things you can do to look after your mind. Some are simple and easy to manage, such as diet and exercise, but others are more complex.

The first thing to realize is that your mind is very sensitive. We don't know the precise factors that contribute to making someone mentally healthy – as always, it seems to be a combination of genetics, environment, habits and life choices – but we know all kinds of things can affect us.

Don't despair if you are diagnosed with a mental health problem

Most of these factors, you won't even notice. Remember, you have limited attention and most of what happens in your mind does so without you noticing (see page 14). While your conscious mind – the thinker – is reflecting on what to say or where to eat later, your automatic mind, the sprinter, is reacting to everything, from internal signals such as feeling hungry or worrying about the future to external factors such as noises, distractions and the other people around you.

You can't control all these factors. All you can do is build good habits, ways of thinking and reacting that help protect your mind from the negative influences around you and give you the energy and perspective to respond well.

Like any area of health, you can't always stay well: your mind is a delicate system and it will sometimes need repairs or maintenance. All you can do is look after yourself, to give yourself the best possible chance of staying well, and recovering quickly.

MENTAL ILLNESS

Even if you lead the most mentally healthy life possible, you can still become mentally unwell. There's no way to eliminate mental illness, but by looking after yourself, staying safe and managing stress you can protect your mind and possibly recover more quickly if you have a problem. By building a mentally healthy routine, you can maximize your chances of staying well, and your hopes for a speedy recovery if you do get sick.

If you are diagnosed with a mental health problem, don't panic: millions of people are diagnosed with mental health issues every year, and the vast majority make full recoveries and manage their conditions well. Being told you have a mental health condition can feel like a life sentence, but things really do get better. Just make sure you seek the right professional help quickly when you need it: your mind is much too important to take chances.

FOOD AND DRINK

Food gives you energy, and since your mind uses energy faster than any other organ, eating healthy, nutritious food can help keep your mind in shape too. Foods that release their energy slowly, such as oatmeal and pulses, can give your mind energy and help you concentrate through the day. Sugary foods have the opposite effect: they do give you more energy in the short term, but you will crash later when the effects wear off, leaving you flat and unable to think straight.

Think about your daily routine: how much energy do you have before and after a meal, and between meals? Are you getting the energy and nutrition you need? Starting your day without food puts pressure on your body, so it's a good idea to eat something in the morning. Breakfast is particularly good for your mind because it helps regulate your sleep patterns, and trains your brain to wake up and eat.

FEED YOUR MIND

Managing what you eat and drink is a great way to improve your mental health. For the most part, feeding your mind is pretty basic: whatever keeps your body healthy also helps keep your mind healthy. There are a few things that particularly help though. Iron, selenium and vitamin D are all good for your mind, so try eating a few brazil nuts, fortified cereals, pulses and seeds such as linseeds and flaxseeds. The brain is 70 percent fat, so fatty acids such as

omega-3 are also useful. You don't need much though, and the effects of these brain-boosting foods are exaggerated. There isn't an easy shortcut to mental health, and as with all these things, it's about finding what works for you.

Many people enjoy a cup of coffee in the morning but beware of depending too much on caffeine and other such substances, as they can become addictive. Caffeine can make you feel more awake, but the more you drink the less alert you will feel without it, until eventually you need coffee just to feel normal. It might even make you feel worse: too much caffeine has been linked to anxiety and tension.

Don't underestimate the impact of diet on your mental state. Think about what you put into your body and how it affects your mind. If you feel anxious, low or tired, the reason may lie in something as simple as what you ate for breakfast.

DIETING AND HUNGER

Controlling what you eat and drink can be tricky though. Dieting takes effort and it's easy to slip into bad habits, eating and drinking things that give us short-term fixes but don't really sustain us. A lot of us end up eating too much and putting on weight, which can affect our self-esteem, lower our mood and cause depression and other psychological health problems.

Hunger is a peculiar thing. It is regulated by your hypothalamus, a basic part of your brain that controls various primal systems. On one level hunger is physical, a sign that your stomach is empty; but it is also psychological, a sense that you haven't had enough to sustain you. Sometimes you can get an impulse to eat when your body doesn't really need it, or crave food that isn't good for you.

This means that dieting can be quite a psychological exercise. Hunger and cravings for food are linked to your emotions and your mood will affect what you want to eat. If you are sad, for example, this depresses your system and can make you feel colder and crave hot, hearty food. Just thinking about food can also make you crave it.

There's even a psychological element to how we perceive food. Research on portion sizes found that we will eat more just because portions are bigger or more food is on offer, so if you want to eat or drink less, buy smaller plates and glasses.

A BALANCED DIET

Our perception of our diet is quite subjective. One study found that people are more likely to eat unhealthy food if they have taken a vitamin pill, while another found that we tend to think foods are healthier if we don't like them, and avoid things that we enjoy because they feel like an indulgence.

As always, try not to get too puritanical about your diet. Build a healthy routine, but make sure you allow yourself a treat once in a while. It's only if the indulgences become routine, or start affecting your health, that you might need to have a word with yourself.

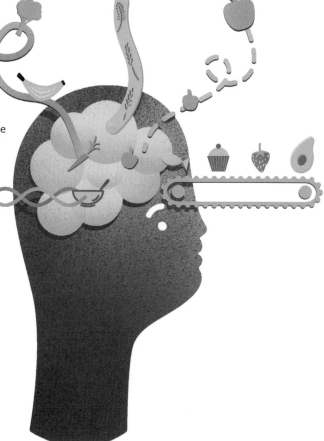

WATER

If you're looking for just one simple thing to do to look after your mind, drink water.

Dehydration is surprisingly bad for your mind. For one thing, it stops you from thinking clearly. Without enough water, it's hard to hold things in your mind or concentrate well, leaving you struggling to make decisions and perform complex tasks.

Water affects your mood too. Even mild dehydration can make you feel tired, tense and anxious. There are also studies that link dehydration to depression. While the effects of dehydration seem to affect women more than men, they do affect all people and not just those who are particularly sensitive or nervous.

In this age of busy lives and skipped lunches, dehydration is still surprisingly common, and you only need to be short by about 500ml (18fl oz) – the equivalent of one small bottle of water – for it to have an effect. So if you're feeling sluggish, flat or struggling to concentrate, drink more water.

HOW MUCH WATER SHOULD YOU DRINK?

You don't need to drink eight glasses of water per day. That's a common guideline, but it doesn't take into account your age, height, weight and other important considerations – such as the water you get from the food you eat. Your mind is pretty good at letting you know when you need to drink more. Do you feel thirsty? Then have a glass of water.

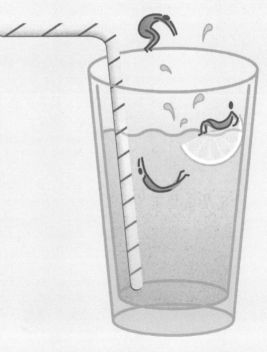

SLEEP

Sleep is really good for our minds. There are lots of theories about the benefits of sleep, from the basic physical effects of resting to more complex theories about the importance of sleep in emotional regulation and memory consolidation. What's certain, though, is that sleep is good.

Going without sleep obviously makes us tired, but it has other effects too. It actually has a similar effect to being drunk, making you woozy and slowing your reactions, which is why you shouldn't drive or operate machinery when you're tired. Lack of sleep can also increase your chances of catching a cold. Getting enough sleep is a wonderful thing, linked to all kinds of benefits including creativity and problem solving, and academic performance. Even an afternoon nap may help you learn.

HOW MUCH SLEEP DO YOU NEED?

A good rule of thumb is that you need one hour of sleep for every two you're awake. Some people can cope with less though, and some need more. We need more sleep when we're younger, probably because our brains keep developing into our twenties, and we may need to sleep less as we get older. It's quite personal. In fact, a 2014 study found you can cope better without sleep if a scientist in a lab coat tells you you've slept enough.

How and when you sleep depends partly on daylight. Natural light during the day regulates your body clock – the background process in your mind that keeps track of your sleep and makes you feel tired at night and awake in the morning. If you spend too much time indoors, without daylight, it can dampen this effect and you can find yourself sleepy during the day or wide awake at 2am. Sunlight also helps your body produce vitamin D, which boosts alertness and general wellbeing.

HOW TO GET A GOOD NIGHT'S SLEEP

What helps you sleep will be quite personal, but below are a few things you can try:

1. Bed means sleep

Many experts say you should design your routine to encourage your mind to sleep when you go to bed. Don't lie in bed working or checking your phone, and if you can't sleep, get out of bed and go somewhere else. Train your mind to know that when you go to bed it's time to go to sleep.

2. Stay somewhere familiar

When you sleep in unfamiliar places you may only be half asleep. A 2016 neuroimaging study suggests half your brain remains awake – keeping watch to make sure it is safe – when you sleep in a new environment. Familiarity is key to sleeping soundly, so develop little rituals such as laying out your clothes and brushing your teeth.

3. Keep warm

A 2009 Dutch study found that small changes in skin temperature affect how well we sleep. A warm bath before bedtime or an electric blanket at night can help keep you sleeping snugly. The researchers even proposed heated sleep suits to keep you warm all night, but maybe try wearing socks first.

4. Put your phone away

Some devices such as mobile phones and tablets produce a kind of blue-white light that our minds think is natural daylight. Being plugged into your phone or laptop all day can make you feel more alert, but then make it harder to switch off later. If you spend a lot of time on your phone at night, what you're effectively doing is telling your brain it is morning, and then asking it to go to sleep. If you're struggling to sleep, turn off the technology half an hour before bedtime.

Don't obsess too much about getting just the right amount of sleep though: worrying about sleep can be counterproductive. Listen to your mind: if you feel like you've had enough sleep, great – but if you don't, well, try not to lose sleep over it.

SLEEP PROBLEMS

Lots of things can get in the way of a good night's sleep. Alcohol, tobacco, medications and even some sleeping pills can make it harder to sleep, and it's hard to relax in a world that is constantly demanding your attention. Insomnia can be a major source of frustration and psychological problems.

It's hard to know how well you're sleeping but if you feel tired, or want to know more about how you sleep, try keeping a sleep diary. Make a note of when you go to sleep and wake up, how you feel in the morning, and anything you remember about your night. You may be surprised by the results. There are also a few apps to help track and improve your sleep too, and the National Sleep Foundation website has many good tips for sleeping well.

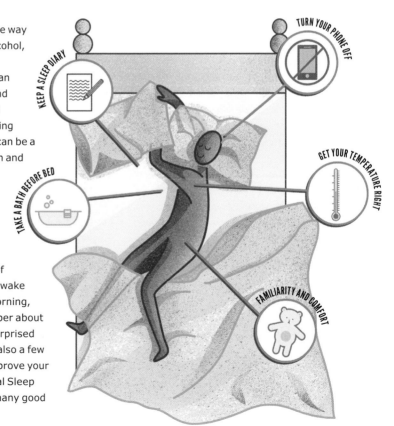

KEEP A SLEEP DIARY

TURN YOUR PHONE OFF

GET YOUR TEMPERATURE RIGHT

TAKE A BATH BEFORE BED

FAMILIARITY AND COMFORT

FITNESS

As your mind is so connected to your body, your physical state will affect your mental and emotional state. Being ill can make you feel sluggish, like that foggy-headed feeling when you're fighting off a cold. Tiredness will have the same effect, and being in physical pain isn't just unpleasant, it's distracting and distressing, leaving you feeling anxious and easily disturbed. Taking care of your body is an excellent way to take care of your mind.

THE BENEFITS OF EXERCISING

Exercise is like a stimulus package for your brain, releasing a cocktail of chemicals that boost mood and raise energy. It reduces activity in areas of the brain associated with worry and depression, and gets your nervous system going. Keeping in good shape can also boost your self-image, regardless of your fitness level.

Vigorous physical exercise such as running, boxing or kung fu can help reduce stress by burning off the excess energy in your mind

and helping you calm down and rest. Exercise doesn't have to be intensive or exhausting though. Even gentle exercise such as going for a walk can help boost your mood and improve your wellbeing, particularly if you do it regularly. Walking in nature is particularly good, walking in a city marginally less so, though it's all pretty personal. Hiking has even been linked with better memory and helping people to avoid some of the negative mental effects of aging.

The key is not to think or talk about exercise, but just to do it

---

GET MOTIVATED

The trouble is, joining a gym is easy, but exercising often isn't. We have good intentions to go running or get to that Pilates class, and then end up sitting on the sofa, watching Netflix and eating snacks. Even if you do get fit, it can be hard to maintain the habit when you have so many other things to do.

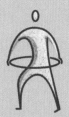
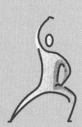
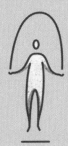
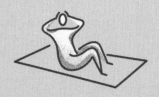

So why is it that our desire to get into shape seems to translate into symbolic gestures more than practical action? There is some evidence that visualizing doing something can reduce your desire to do it. In one study, thirsty people were encouraged to visualize drinking a cool glass of water, but this actually made them feel less thirsty, even though they were still just as dehydrated. This is why watching sport is so fun: you can have all the virtuous feelings of a workout without leaving your sofa.

The key then, is not to think or talk about exercise, but just to do it. So the real question is what is the simplest sort of exercise you can take right now? You don't have to join a gym or take up mountaineering: just walk up the stairs, run on the spot, do some sit-ups or lift a chair a few times. Do whatever you can to get the daily habit of taking a little exercise – and when you find the chair is too light for you, or you get bored of running on the carpet, join a gym. You can get a lot of exercise just by changing your routine a little.

PRESSURE TO BE PERFECT

One of the biggest motivators for taking up exercise is wanting to be more like the slender, toned people on the television and in magazines.

Be careful with this though: exercise, like dieting, can become an addiction, and you can end up chasing the perfect body to the detriment of your peace of mind. One study on gym habits found that putting mirrors in a gym made people more demoralized and less active. Even people who were happy with their appearance were affected.

Real fitness isn't about being the right dress size or lifting more than your friends. It's about keeping your body active, keeping your heart, lungs and other key systems in good working order, and having enough energy to do the things you want.

 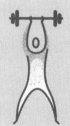  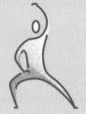

HEALTHY HABITS

Very often, we know what's good for us. We set goals and resolutions to eat better or exercise more, but somehow our minds let us down. This is another reason why it is so important to consider mental health alongside physical health.

We need to get much better at recognizing the psychological components in many public health issues. Smoking, addictions, obesity, drug abuse, even less dangerous addictions such as retail therapy and obsessive gaming are all, at their core, methods for managing how we feel. The more we use such ineffective, destructive tools to self-manage, the worse our collective health gets. Yet swap these destructive habits for something healthier and more sustainable and you may start to notice that your health, both physical and mental, improves.

GOOD AND BAD HABITS

Psychologists now study health habits. People who engage in "protective habits", such as sleeping well and exercising regularly, tend to have fewer illnesses, longer life expectancy and higher wellbeing. On the other side, bad habits such as smoking, drinking, working long hours or eating unhealthily can damage your health.

Most of us are taught good heath habits as kids, learning to brush our teeth, wash our hands and so on. The trouble is, we learn bad habits too. Both come easily to us. The problem is that changing your bad habits is hard work.

CHANGING HABITS

A habit is a type of memory in which the automatic part of your mind (the sprinter, see page 14) recalls a successful strategy that it's tried before, and does it again, saving you time and energy.

You can retrain your habits using your thinker (see page 15), by consciously interrupting your routine and training yourself to respond differently. This takes work though: remember, your thinker uses energy faster than your sprinter, so it is tiring constantly watching yourself and checking your behaviour. Once the habit is formed, though, it becomes automatic and easy again.

In his book *The Power of Habit*, the investigative reporter Charles Duhigg argues that you can change your habits by understanding how they are triggered, and what benefit you get from them.

A habit is made up of a cue, a routine and a reward. There is a situation that triggers the habit, the habitual behaviour itself, and a reward at the end, the material or psychological benefit you gain from it. If the reward is particularly strong, you remember the habit more quickly.

According to Duhigg, the golden rule of habit change is simple: if you keep the same cue and the same reward, you can change the habit in the middle. Let's say you want to stop smoking, for example. Here's how it works:

1. Notice when you do it

Figure out what prompts you to want to smoke. Are there particular times of the day or situations that increase the craving, such as being out with friends or being stressed at work? Notice what prompts you to want to smoke, because these are the moments when you need to be extra vigilant.

2. Understand the benefit

There might be an obvious thing you gain from smoking, but it might also be more complicated than you think. Many people say they smoke to calm down, but it could also be about being sociable with your friends, or a feeling of rebellion. Figure out what you gain from it, why you like it.

3. Find a new habit instead

When you feel the urge to smoke, you need to replace this routine with something else that gives you the same reward. If you smoke to calm down, find another way to relax instead.

If you smoke to be sociable, practise other ways of having fun with friends. Find something you enjoy as much as smoking – that isn't as bad for you – and do that instead.

OLD HABITS DIE HARD

All this takes effort of course, and there will be times when you fall back into old patterns, particularly when you are tired or stressed. It gets easier though. The more you practise, the less energy it takes. There's even some evidence that exercising self-discipline is itself a habit – so the more you change your habits, the better you get at it.

Habits are automatic loops that your sprinter uses to respond quickly to situations. There is a cue that triggers it, a routine response, and a resulting reward. Your thinker can retrain your sprinter to respond differently, but it takes effort.

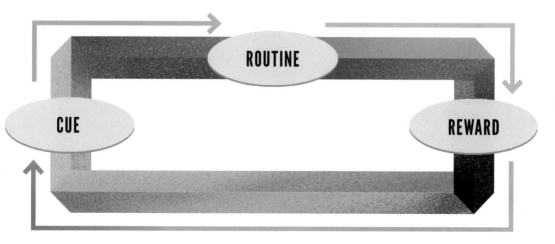

SOCIALIZING

Looking after your mind can feel like a solitary activity at times, fighting off temptation, trying to eat well and hitting the treadmill. But mental health is much more varied than physical health, and one of the biggest influences on our state of mind is the people around us.

Socializing is very important for a healthy mind. Social contact has been linked to all sorts of health and wellbeing factors, including reduced stress, better physical health and lower mortality. One review even concluded that loneliness could take as many years off your life expectancy as smoking, alcohol and obesity.

Absorbing yourself in an activity can be great for improving your mood, but it's even better if you do it with other people. The opposite of this, feeling useless and forgotten, is extremely bad, which may explain why retirement and unemployment can be so bad for people's mental health.

Other people are incredibly important for our mental health

Sometimes the source of how you feel is not in your own mind, but in the minds of the people around you (see page 145). Happy people can make you feel happier, anxious people can make you more anxious.

NOT ALL SOCIAL CONTACT IS GOOD FOR US

Sometimes other people can make us feel worse. Bullying and discrimination are very bad for our minds, and many mental health problems are associated with being disadvantaged, attacked or otherwise being on the wrong side of society. Feeling unsafe is also very bad for us, and there is a wealth of studies linking mental illness to violent crime, social exclusion, poverty and disadvantage.

Sometimes you need to engage with unpleasant or aggressive people, but don't seek them out for the sake of it: your mind will be much better for their absence.

People can be sources of stress and annoyance but, all in all, other people are incredibly important for our mental health. Investing in relationships and spending time with people you like are central to a healthy way of life. If you feel flat or unhappy, talk to someone: it's amazing how it can bring you out of yourself.

MINDAPPLES

A healthy, well-fed, relaxed mind is the best asset you can have, but how you get there is personal to you. So the question you need to ask yourself is a simple one: what do you do that's good for your mind?

Since 2008, the Mindapples campaign has been asking people this question (see pages 6–7). A "mindapple" is anything you do to look after your mind. It could be one of the healthy habits listed in this chapter, such as drinking water or taking exercise, but your mind is unique to you, and it doesn't lend itself quite as easily to one-size-fits-all solutions.

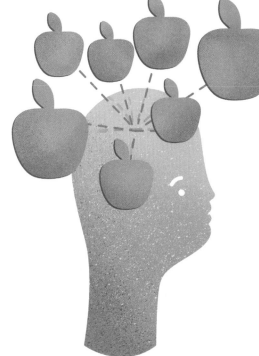

HAVING FUN IS GOOD FOR YOU

Research by the psychologist Sarah Pressman and her colleagues in 2009 found that while there are some obvious things we can all do to look after our minds, what is much more important is finding enjoyable healthy activities that fit your way of life. They found that people who spend more time doing things they enjoy tend to be happier, like their lives more, suffer less depression and stress, have lower blood pressure and enjoy better physical health.

Taking time out to relax can serve as a "breather", a chance to take a break and distract oneself from the demands and concerns that occupy the mind. Leisure activities can also act as "restorers", helping us cope with stress and adversity by replenishing our resources. So, while it might not feel quite as virtuous as quitting smoking or getting an early night, it seems you really can take care of your health by doing things you enjoy.

This explains why the list of things that are apparently good for our minds is so ridiculously long. There are health benefits to art and music, but that doesn't mean everyone likes going to galleries, or likes the same songs. Hugging is good for your wellbeing, but being forced to hug each other is not. Retail therapy can cheer you up, but don't expect your doctor to prescribe you more time on eBay. There is even a study that says watching *The Lord of the Rings* is good for reducing depression – but only if you like *The Lord of the Rings*.

When it comes to our day-to-day wellbeing, prescriptive approaches are pretty limited.

Instead, each of us needs to think about what our mind needs, then share it with others, and talk about it together.

WHAT ARE YOUR MINDAPPLES?

So you can take care of your physical health by going for a run, or eating an apple, but what is the equivalent for your mental health? What is the 5-a-day for your mind? Thousands of people all around the world have now shared their mindapples, and this book is peppered with a small selection of their suggestions (*see opposite*, for example). As you will see, there isn't an obvious pattern to what people do for their minds; the answers are very personal, from yoga to karaoke, going out dancing to polishing furniture.

Some of the mindapples cover the basics, such as getting exercise or eating healthily, but there are some pretty sophisticated techniques out there too. People talk about how they practise being grateful for what they have or getting perspective on their problems. Some people meditate or go running, others play golf or read the Bible.

So what are your mindapples? Think about what you do every day, or regularly, to look after your mind. They can be anything you like. It's your mind.

MAKE TIME FOR YOUR MIND

Make time in your day for the things that make you feel calm and happy. It may feel more important in the moment to cross off an extra thing from your to-do list, or to help out a friend or family member, but if you neglect your mental health and wellbeing then you will struggle to get things done, and be no use to anyone else. Give yourself permission to manage your mind: your health, and your life will improve.

Make time for whatever "breathers" and "restorers" you enjoy, and try to develop lasting habits to keep your mind in good condition. You rely on your mind for everything you do, so look after it.

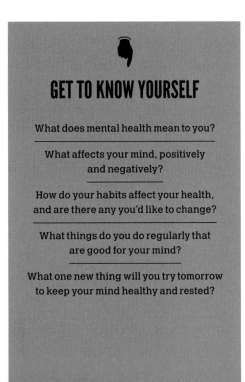

GET TO KNOW YOURSELF

What does mental health mean to you?

What affects your mind, positively and negatively?

How do your habits affect your health, and are there any you'd like to change?

What things do you do regularly that are good for your mind?

What one new thing will you try tomorrow to keep your mind healthy and rested?

WHAT WORKS FOR YOU?

Feel grass under my feet.

Stretch my body like a cat.

Take a proper lunch break.

Get at least 7 hours' sleep a night.

Always carry a bottle of water.

HOW
TO
BE
WISE

YOUR AMAZING BRAIN

The human brain is the most remarkable system we've ever found in nature. Although many of its secrets still elude us, what we do know is astounding.

Our brains can perform trillions of operations per second and hold thousands of terabytes of information, all in a compressed space and at very low power. The human brain contains approximately 86 billion neurons, according to the neuroanatomist Suzana Herculano-Houzel, yet it weighs about the same as a toaster. As technology goes, your brain is the most powerful gadget you will ever own.

LEARNING HOW TO THINK

The trouble is, our brains are also a little bit stupid. We get stuck in unhelpful loops, struggle to remember things, fail to explain ourselves and make obvious, avoidable mistakes. Some people seem to be wiser than the rest of us, but even the cleverest person can be fooled.

To understand why, we need to look at how our brains evolved. Over the past 100,000 years, our brains have been adapting to the challenges around us, changing from animal brains into something a bit different. We may drive cars and work in offices now, but we have the brains of hunter-gatherers. In fact, our primitive ancestors may even have been smarter than us: the intellectual demands of gathering food and tracking animals are higher than the average office job, which may explain why Neanderthals appear to have had larger brains than we do today.

So the starting point for becoming wise is to understand your mind. To make smart choices and have good opinions, you need to understand how you think, when to trust your instincts and when to check your reasoning. Without the humility to question your thinking, you can never learn to think better. To be smart, you must first realize that you are stupid.

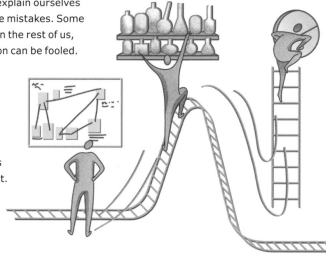

THOUGHTLESSNESS

One of the amazing things about your mind is how much you can do without really thinking. You make most of your daily choices automatically, and the vast majority are absolutely right.

This is because our minds have evolved to take action, not to overthink things. As the cognitive scientist Tom Stafford argues in his excellent book *For Argument's Sake*, human reason is defined by the need to act, not pure logic. We get up, get dressed, go out, come home and go to bed, all with minimal effort and few errors. Your mind evolved for getting things done, not getting things right.

THE SPRINTER
These everyday decisions are handled by the automatic part of your mind, the sprinter (see page 14). The sprinter leaps into action first, remembering past choices, deciding quickly and handling familiar activities. The sprinter does almost all your thinking, and it is always needed, always running.

Your sprinter can dart all over the place, spotting connections, noticing similarities and coming to quick conclusions. In fact, most of our decisions never even make it to our conscious awareness. For example, classic experiments at the University of Iowa found that gamblers react to risks unconsciously before they notice them consciously. This is what we mean by "gut feelings" or intuition. You don't think things through and then take action: you act first, and think later.

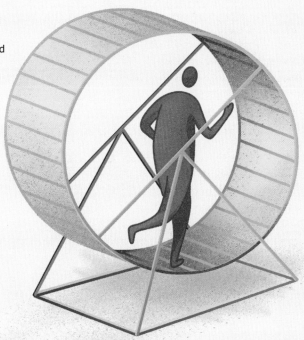

THE THINKER

Your second response, the thinker (see page 15), comes into play when you need to reflect on your first response and perhaps change your mind. The thinker is methodical and analytical, and it can use tools too – write things down, draw diagrams, discuss ideas and use technology to tackle problems that are too complex for the sprinter.

The trouble is, you don't always use your thinker to think things through objectively: instead, you may use it to justify your original choice, entrench your position and defend your image. Even when you choose to think things through in a more controlled way, your automatic reactions are still there in the background, influencing your thinking. As the educational psychologist David Perkins at Harvard argues, many of our opinions are essentially thoughtless. We form a first impression, then look for evidence to support it, and if we find it, we stop thinking. Counter-evidence is then dismissed, often without ever being considered.

This is the thinker's curse: it comes too late to the party, after the matter has already been decided. Instead of using our minds to get things right, we use them to justify being wrong.

WISE MINDS

These, then, are the tools we use to make all of our decisions. A sprinter that is prone to errors, and a thinker that is unduly influenced by its unreliable partner. By learning how your mind forms opinions and comes to conclusions, you can be more thoughtful, reduce the risk of errors and get more decisions right.

There are two areas where you can improve on how you think:

- **Training your sprinter, to improve your first responses and making your intuition more reliable.**
- **Strengthening your thinker, to think things through more carefully and to spot more mistakes.**

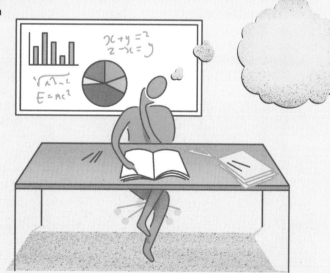

USE YOUR HEAD

mindapples

TRAINING YOUR SPRINTER

Whenever you encounter a situation, your mind tries to connect it to things it's seen before. If the situation is familiar, such as crossing a road or meeting a friend, you may repeat what you did last time. If it is unfamiliar, you will often try to find a template to help you make sense of the situation and take action.

These associations don't follow logical paths, but are shaped by a network of implicit associations: knowledge and experiences, stories you've heard, things you imagined, irrelevant features such as shapes and colours, and even what other people think. Your mind puts all these things together and you get a good or a bad feeling about something. You can't tell where this intuition has come from, so you can't be sure whether it's right. In fact, the job of the sprinter is to be overconfident: it keeps you moving with purpose, even when you are lost.

IMPROVING YOUR FIRST RESPONSE

The more accurate, relevant associations you have for a topic, the better your mind can tackle the situation. The way to improve your first response is through learning – expanding your experiences and building more accurate associations, training your mind to respond in smarter ways.

Let's say you want to get to know the property market. At first you have to do everything by the book, listing features, comparing prices and listening to expert advice. But after a while, you start to get a sense of it. Your intuition improves and you get good feelings about places that are well priced, or that will suit your needs. After early uncertainty, your sprinter slowly learns the ropes, until you go from judging places by the colour of the curtains to saying meaningful things about square footage and market value.

The job of the sprinter is to be overconfident: it keeps you moving, even when you are lost

---

In simple terms, the more you know about a subject, the more you can trust your intuition. In other words, you need to become an expert.

Gaining expertise is incredibly useful. In order to know if you should trust your instinct (or someone else's, for that matter), you need to know if that instinct is informed by expertise, or if it is just a wayward sprinter being overconfident again.

HOW TO BE AN EXPERT

Learning is a complex subject, but if you want to acquire expertise in a field, there are a few useful tricks to bear in mind.

BREAK THINGS DOWN

We learn in small chunks, so don't overload your mind. Learn one thing, then the next, breaking things down into micro-steps and giving your mind time to absorb each one. Our memories may even specialize too, so the more things you learn about a topic, the easier it gets to remember what you've learned.

PAY ATTENTION

In her book *Mastermind: How to Think Like Sherlock Holmes*, writer and psychologist Maria Konnikova argues that the key to learning is "memory encoding" – filing your memories carefully in your mental library. The more you pay attention, the better you encode memories. Avoid distractions and train your mind to focus on one thing, and you should find the things you learn become easier to recall.

DISCUSS WHAT YOU'VE LEARNED

When you recall a memory, you make it stronger and easier to remember, so explaining a topic or retelling a story can help you remember those things better. Remembering one thing makes it easier to remember other things too, so the more you connect your knowledge together, the easier it gets to remember what you know.

LOOK AFTER YOUR MIND

Your mind is the tool you're using for all this, so keep it well fed, focused and free from stress and distractions. Sleeping after learning something can help you remember it later, and being in a positive mood might help you absorb information better, while stress is very bad for learning. Spending time in nature seems to help too, as well as doing hobbies and other things you enjoy.

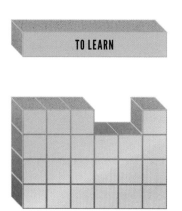

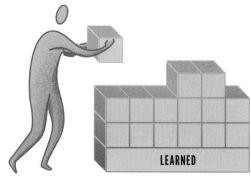

WATCHING YOUR MIND

Even the most energetic mind is still vulnerable to mistakes. Your automatic mind relies on simple rules to make quick choices and get you through the day. These rules are often called unconscious biases.

We aren't aware of these biases, but they affect our minds in oddly consistent ways. By watching your mind and remembering how it can be fooled, you can reduce at least some of the negative effects of these biases on your thinking.

WHAT ARE YOUR UNCONSCIOUS BIASES?

There are dozens of biases that could be affecting you. You don't need to remember them all, but here are some of the most common. How many can you spot in yourself?

🍎 We are selective with evidence
- We fixate on one piece of information and ignore others.
- We assign more importance to information that's easy to remember.
- We remember unusual things better than commonplace things.
- We look for evidence that agrees with our opinions, and reject the rest.
- We continue to be influenced by evidence after we find out it is false.

🍎 We are too proud
- We think we are less biased than other people for no good reason.
- We overestimate our knowledge, capabilities and level of control.
- We think we made better choices in the past than we actually did.
- We ignore valid information just because we don't like who said it.

🍎 We are easily led
- We do things that everyone else does without questioning.
- We make different decisions depending on context and presentation.
- We like things just because they seem familiar to us.
- We notice what's in front of us, but don't notice when things are missing.

🍎 We stand by our mistakes
- We respond to counter-evidence by becoming even more entrenched in our views.
- We throw more resources into bad decisions rather than cutting our losses.
- We take big risks to avoid losses, but not to achieve gains.
- We make up false reasons for our choices in hindsight.

🍎 We are bad at prioritizing
- We focus on trivial decisions and ignore important decisions.
- We favour smaller short-term gains over greater long-term ones.
- We are more worried about losing what we have than gaining new things.
- We focus on the costs of taking action, rather than not taking action.

We suck at probability

- We ignore risks and pretend things are certain when they aren't.
- We think specific predictions are more likely than vague predictions.
- We think things become less likely if they've happened recently.
- We think bad things are unlikely to happen, and good things are likely.

We see patterns everywhere

- We personify abstract forces and see intention behind random events.
- We think there are connections between things that are coincidental.
- We notice things more when we heard about them recently.
- We find statements to be more believable if they rhyme.

CORRECTING FOR BIAS

No one ever thinks they're being biased, of course. We rarely admit to being gullible or easily influenced. In fact, we are excellent at inventing plausible reasons for our decisions, to pretend we are more rational than we are.

Because of this, correcting for all these biases isn't easy; no one can escape influences all the time. With practice, though, you can become more aware of the patterns in your thinking, and correct for them – particularly for very important decisions. Perhaps this is why, in a recent study on improving people's decision-making, the most effective thing to do was study psychology.

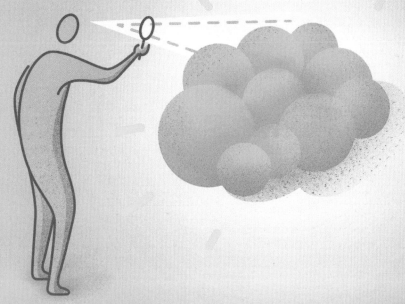

RETRAINING YOUR MIND

This process of retraining your mind works for attitudes too. Your automatic mind is full of opinions about subjects of which you know very little. You make pre-judgments, before you know the facts, and are often wrong.

Harvard's Project Implicit spent years mapping these implicit associations that afflict us all, which include fear of other races, gender stereotyping, mistrust of foreigners, and many other unhelpful things. We get these stereotypes from the media, the people around us and our own experiences. We're all susceptible, regardless of who we are or where we come from.

every response, is training your mind, so try to expose yourself to intelligent, educated input rather than bombarding your brain with fake news and advertising. When it comes to your unconscious mind, you get out what you put in.

Familiarity doesn't breed contempt; it destroys it

These associations can be changed though. We tend to be wary of unfamiliar things, but get comfortable once we know something is safe, moving from an instinct to avoid to an instinct to approach. This is called the exposure effect. The more you see foreign words, the more you like hearing them. Areas with high immigration tend to be more positive about immigrants. Familiarity doesn't breed contempt; it destroys it. (This is how advertising works too: the more you see a brand, the more you are drawn to it.)

So generally, the more experience you have, the more you can trust your judgment. Bear in mind though, that every bit of input,

CHECK YOUR THINKING

Since most of the decisions you make happen without you noticing, you need to make an effort to notice when you have leaped to a false conclusion, and ask yourself what has influenced your choice. Are you responding to the facts, or something else?

This process of checking your thinking takes energy. Remember, your thinker uses more energy than your sprinter, so correcting for biases takes more effort than acting on instinct. It's important to make the effort, though, or else you can end up making mistakes, treating people badly and believing all kinds of stupid things.

GETTING CLEAR ON THE FACTS

The philosopher Bertrand Russell, in his advice to the next generation, said that whatever you're trying to do, first you must get clear on the facts, and the truth that those facts bear out.

A great many of the problems that afflict our lives, from poor life choices to falling out with our friends, stem from a lack of understanding of the facts. If you don't know what's going on, responding effectively is going to be tricky.

HOW CAN YOU KNOW WHAT'S TRUE?

For thousands of years, philosophers have been arguing about the underlying principles of knowledge. There aren't any easy answers, but there are a few obvious ways to check what we know.

The most obvious starting point is your own experience. After all, if you can't trust your own eyes, what can you trust? The trouble is, our minds aren't very good at distinguishing between fact and fiction. What happens in your brain is quite similar for experiencing something and imagining something, so it can be hard to separate what happened from what you think happened.

Memory can be unreliable too: you don't recall things as accurately as you think, and the more you retell facts and stories, the more your memories of them can change. Eyewitness testimony is notoriously unreliable, and people often have vivid memories of things that didn't happen to them.

For this reason, you often also need to use logic, thinking experiences through and applying deductive reasoning to assess them and form conclusions. The trouble is, logic is difficult, and it's hard to be sure whether your reasoning is sound. Many intelligent people have come to false conclusions because they missed a crucial piece of evidence or made a mistake in their reasoning. In fact, a study in 2015 found that professional philosophers were just as biased and irrational as the rest of us. Reason can be an unreliable master.

TESTING YOUR IDEAS

Most of the time, we don't rely on our own experiences or reasoning, but on those of the

BE INFORMED, NOT OPINIONATED

The US investor Charlie Munger argues that you should never disagree with someone unless you know more about the subject than they do. In his 1995 talk at Harvard, The Psychology of Human Misjudgment, he advocated that people should try to be informed, rather than opinionated. Having an opinion is easy; having an informed opinion takes work. Think through your opinions and figure out what facts need to be true for you to be right. If the main reason you hold an opinion is because you want it to be true, you may need to reconsider.

people around us. The world is too complicated to master everything yourself: you need to take things on faith. If everyone can see a glass on the table, there's probably a glass on the table. If you can see it, but your friend can't, you may be seeing things. This is how science works too. Scientific experiments are designed to be repeatable, so researchers can check each other's findings. If no one else can repeat your findings, your theory is less reliable. (This is currently a big problem in psychology.)

With so much information now available to us, the importance of knowing who and what to trust has never been more difficult. Philosopher A C Grayling, speaking at the 2015 Festival of Dangerous Ideas in Sydney, argued that what we need to learn today is how to be good evaluators of information, critical assessors of what we read and hear.

Our minds aren't naturally very good at following logical processes, so here are a few principles from philosophy that can help you assess the quality of an idea:

1. Set aside your prejudices

Try to look at the evidence objectively and focus on what is true, not what you wish to be true or think would be good. Question your assumptions, and ask yourself what you want the answer to be, and try to bracket out those desires in your analysis. Approaching the world in a non-judgmental way is great for making good decisions.

2. Keep things simple

One of the big tricks our minds play on us is inventing complex explanations for simple problems. The classic antidote to this is Occam's razor, named after the 14th-century philosopher William of Occam. If two explanations seem equally plausible, choose the simplest one. Indeed, one of the symptoms

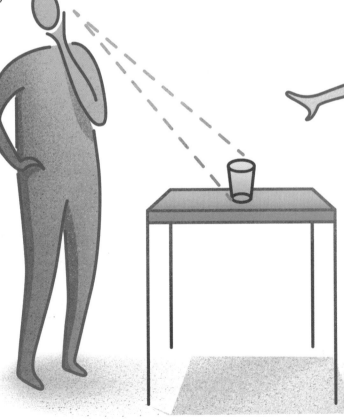

of delusional thinking is inventing more and more complex explanations to make your theory work. Ask yourself: how many things need to be true for your theory to be right?

3. Understand causality
Most factual arguments are based on causality: the idea that one thing caused another. This sounds simple enough, but we are surprisingly bad at it. Firstly, we often get it the wrong way around, thinking that because one thing caused another, this means the reverse is true too. The most famous example of this is cargo cults: Pacific islanders who thought that because cargo planes landed on airstrips during World War II, they could make more planes land by recreating these airstrips. Secondly, we mistake correlation (two things happening together) for causation (one thing happening because of another thing). The two things might both be caused by an unrelated event, or be completely unconnected.

4. Think it through
We are prone to what psychologists call the illusion of explanatory depth. We think we understand things because we know a little bit about them, but our thinking unravels when questioned. Just because you have googled something, it doesn't mean that you know more about it than an expert. Explain your theory, step by step, without any gaps, and you may discover that there is more to consider than you first thought.

KNOW WHEN YOU'RE WRONG
One of the key ideas in the history of science is the concept of falsification. The philosopher Karl Popper proposed that theories are only useful if they can be disproved – if there are things that could render your argument false. Don't just think about what needs to be true for your theory to work: think about why it wouldn't work. Figure out what would convince you that you are wrong, and test it out. If you try to disprove your theory, and fail, it's more likely to be right.

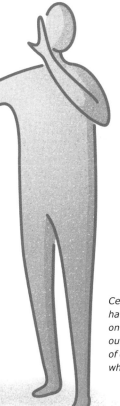

Certainty is a luxury we rarely have, so instead, we must rely on all kinds of clues, such as our own senses or the views of other people, to figure out what is really going on.

THE ART OF PROBABILITY

There is rarely such a thing as an ideal decision or a perfect opinion. Ideas that look right at the time can turn out to be wrong. The truth is, as a species, we are uncertain.

The arguments of the Sceptics of Ancient Greece are still hard to refute. All your knowledge is based on your experiences, and ultimately all these experiences could be in your imagination – the creation of an evil demon, as the French philosopher René Descartes put it. The cloud of unknowing follows us everywhere.

But this doesn't mean you should give up. You have to put your faith in something. The key is not to strive for the right answer. Instead, think about which option is probably right. This may seem obvious, but it is a surprisingly recent approach to logic and wisdom.

NOTHING IS CERTAIN
The philosopher Ian Hacking, in his book *The Emergence of Probability*, argues that one of the key moments in the history of ideas was the creation of probability theory, the quantification of our uncertainty. Thinking in probabilities doesn't come naturally to us. Our minds love certainty – we decide if things are true and then move on. Fuzziness and complexity are tiring and stressful. If you want to be smart though, you need to accept that nothing is certain.

There is a lot of pressure on us to have opinions about everything these days, from trade policy to climate change. But resist. It's perfectly respectable to say you don't know enough, and put your trust in others instead. In fact, the wisest line attributed to Socrates, the founder of Classical philosophy, is that he knew that he knew nothing.

The writer Christopher Hitchens used to say that the quality of your mind is not determined by what you think, but by how you think. Thinking is not a skill with which we are born, but a discipline to be practised.

Pay attention to your instincts, build up your expertise, focus your mental energy, watch for biases, and keep thinking about the possibilities you might have missed, and you will increase your chances of being wise.

GET TO KNOW YOURSELF

What decisions do you make during a typical day, and how do you make them?

What are the biggest mistakes you've made in the past, and why did they seem right at the time?

What biases do you particularly need to watch out for in your thinking?

How can you check your thinking and get clear on the facts of each situation?

What do you have faith in, and why?

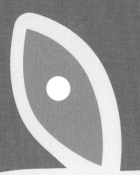

WHAT WORKS FOR YOU?

Check knowledge - am I thinking straight?

Read for 10-15 minutes before bed.

Try something new - learn Chinese.

Argument and debate.

Rest.

HOW TO BE PRODUCTIVE

HOW TO BE PRODUCTIVE

BETTER, FASTER, STRONGER

Productivity is big business. Flip through the pages of business books and magazines and you will find a dizzying array of tips and techniques for getting more done.

Productivity is only a means to an end though. Doing things quickly is good, but only if you're doing the right things. It's not about quantity, but quality; about being effective. Whatever your goal, whether it's to get promoted, spend more time with your family or pass your exams, it's useful to know how to apply your mind effectively to the challenges facing you.

IMPROVING YOUR PRODUCTIVITY

Most productivity tips claim to be universal rules for getting things done, but in fact many are specific to a particular activity or profession. Productivity is not one unified discipline: techniques often work for one kind of task but not for others.

Somewhere in the midst of all the advice, though, there is a simple but important question: what helps your mind perform at its best? Which factors can help you get your mind into the best possible shape to think and work, and apply it effectively to your to-do list?

Thanks to decades of research into management theory, cognition, attention, learning and many other areas, we can offer

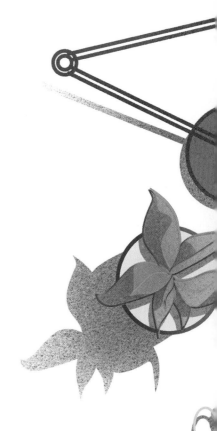

a few answers to this question. Everyone is different though, so the specific techniques you use to achieve these things will be personal to you. But based on the literature and what people say works for them, there are a few principles of productivity that can help you achieve more with your time, and waste less.

Many of these principles are easy to explain, but hard to do. Productivity takes discipline, at least at first, and you won't transform your level

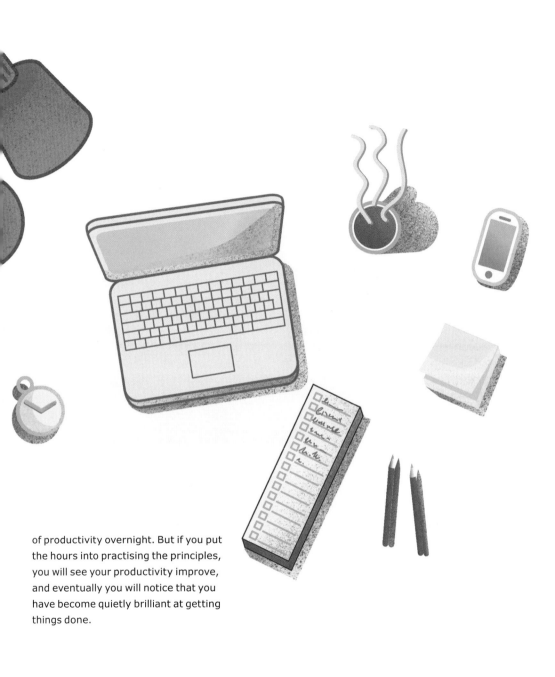

of productivity overnight. But if you put the hours into practising the principles, you will see your productivity improve, and eventually you will notice that you have become quietly brilliant at getting things done.

GET MOTIVATED

Productivity is all about application. However smart or knowledgeable you are, you won't get very far unless you can apply your mind to what you're doing. The trouble is, it's pretty hard to force yourself to do things you don't want to do. Continually reminding yourself why you need to do something takes energy – energy that could be better spent on getting things done.

What you really want is to reach a state where you don't need to force yourself, and action feels easy. We call this state of productive energy "motivation". It isn't an intellectual process, but an emotional one, a feeling of flow and excitement. It is your most engaged and productive state.

Finding your motivation is the first principle of productivity. The research of psychologists such as Marylène Gagné, Edward Deci and Hugo Kehr has identified a number of factors that, together, seem to get people motivated:

- An incentive to act.
- A personal connection to the task.
- The belief that you will succeed.

WHY NOW?

We all need an incentive to do things. These external or "extrinsic" motivators come from outside you, pulling you into action. They can be positive, such as a financial reward or prize, and they can be negative, such as avoiding a fine or protecting your assets: the carrot and the stick.

The importance of external incentives depends on the task. For repetitive tasks that don't take much thought, we tend to need incentives to do them because they are dull. For more interesting or creative tasks, though, too much focus on external incentives can make us do less, not more.

In classic experiments by Deci in the 1970s, some people were paid to do puzzles, while others were given nothing. Surprisingly, the unpaid participants did more work and solved more puzzles, even though they had less incentive to do so. The same was true of negative incentives too. When people were criticized or fined if they failed, they too did the minimum. The addition of incentives made an interesting task feel boring.

Money is still important though. Worrying about money can distract and demoralize you, and you need to feel fairly compensated or you may become resentful. But beyond that, more money doesn't seem to produce more effort.

Incentives are mainly useful, because they provide urgency. Without an immediate incentive, you can still like a task, but you won't necessarily make time for it.

WHY ME?

Whether we employ the carrot or the stick method, external incentives are not enough to motivate people on their own. You also need a personal connection to the task, a feeling that it is the right thing for you to do yourself.

Internal or "intrinsic" motivators come from within you, from your values, beliefs and desires. They push you into action.

These higher causes lead us to work harder and go the extra mile. We are very motivated by relationships too, so doing things for other people is often more motivating than doing them for yourself. On the other side, you will be less willing to do something if you know it will cause problems for other people, or affect how much they like you.

Internal incentives don't have to be worthy: sometimes you want to do something because you enjoy doing it. It may just feel like your thing, something personal to you that you can do your way. That sense of autonomy and control is a key part of feeling enthusiastic about an activity.

Intrinsic motivators are particularly important for creative or analytic tasks. You can have all the incentives you like to be brilliant, but unless you have that inner drive, you will struggle to apply the whole of your mind to the task at hand.

Without an inner connection to the task, we tend to do the minimum and work to rule. This has been a priority for many businesses in recent years: simply paying people for their work is fine if they don't need to use their brains, but in the knowledge economy, staff engagement is the key to productivity.

HOW CAN I SUCCEED?

The final ingredient of motivation is the one we most often forget. You can have all the incentives and passion for something you like, but unless you feel able to do it, you will get stuck. The belief that you can succeed is key.

Your belief in your ability depends partly on the skills and resources you can bring to the task. If you know how to do it, or know someone who can, then it feels achievable. This is where knowledge and experience come in. Things can feel daunting at first, but once you've done them they feel more manageable. Money and physical assets help here too, but they aren't everything, so don't fixate on them.

We tend to be more motivated to do things we're good at. Seeing your abilities improve is particularly motivating: studies by the psychologist Carol Dweck showed that people who attribute their successes to hard work, rather than innate talent, are more likely to succeed.

This doesn't mean things need to be easy. We all like a challenge, and if a task is too easy you may not give it your full attention. Rising to challenges and stretching our abilities make us feel good, and can increase our abilities too. The optimum level of challenge is when a task uses the full extent of your abilities. The more you push yourself, the more motivated you can become.

LEARN TO CONCENTRATE

Multitasking is making us crazy. Constant interruptions, too much information and the constant beep of smartphones: the modern world can be pretty destructive to our peace of mind. With so many things competing for our attention, the second principle of productivity is focusing your mind.

In truth, though, you aren't really multitasking. All your mind can do is switch quickly from one task to the next, creating the impression that you're doing them simultaneously. We can get pretty good at this task-switching, but it comes at a cost: every time you switch your attention you deplete your mental energy. Switch all the time, and you can end up slow and sluggish. In fact, a 2013 study found heavy multitaskers scored lower in IQ tests.

FOCUS YOUR ATTENTION ON ONE THING AT A TIME

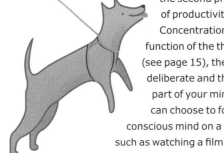

Learning to concentrate is the second principle of productivity. Concentration is a function of the thinker (see page 15), the deliberate and thoughtful part of your mind. You can choose to focus your conscious mind on a task, such as watching a film

or thinking about a particularly tough problem, and everything else seems to fade into the background, a bit like moving a mental spotlight.

In fact, we are so good at concentrating on one thing that we can miss obvious things around us. One famous attention experiment asked people to count basketball throws and showed how our minds are so good at tuning out our surroundings that we can lose all awareness of what's happening. (If you haven't seen this experiment, search for "Simons' selective attention test" online and try the game yourself.)

The trouble is, you can also have your attention pulled elsewhere, drawn to something nearby, such as a movement or a sound, or remembering something you'd forgotten. These distractions interrupt your "top-down" focus and take you away from what you were trying to do.

According to the cognitive psychologists Maurizio Corbetta and Gordon Shulman, this type of "bottom-up" attention is actually a separate system, and uses a different part of your brain. You can put your attention on one thing, but then find it grabbed by something else. There is one pathway for concentration, another for distraction. The main purpose of this second attention system is to keep you safe. You can be absorbed in a task, but your mind is still scanning for threats.

The skill of concentration, then, is not to allow your focused attention to be interrupted by these distractions. You need to strengthen the system for focus, and calm the system for watching your surroundings.

HOW TO IMPROVE YOUR CONCENTRATION

There are a lot of different techniques for improving your concentration skills, but a few seem to be particularly beneficial:

1. Control your surroundings

The simplest way to avoid distraction is to simplify your surroundings and minimize the number of things that can attract your attention. Loud or erratic noises can pull you out of what you're doing, and so can distracting movements. The main problem is not the distractions themselves though (the background hum of a coffee shop can aid creativity, for example), it's being surrounded by things beyond your control. If you can't control your environment, you may feel helpless and vulnerable, which heightens your awareness. If you feel unsafe, your mind watches for threats, and you can't focus on what you're doing.

2. Manage your moods

Not all distractions are external. Memories and feelings, particularly negative ones, can interrupt your concentration. Try to deal with difficult emotions and avoid worries. If your mind is free from these inner preoccupations, you can focus more brainpower on what you are doing.

3. Stay fresh

It's much harder to tune out distractions when you're tired. Get plenty of sleep, eat well and avoid short-term boosts such as sugary foods and energy drinks. For sustained attention, you need to look after your mind.

4. Meditate

The best way we know to train attention is mindfulness meditation (see page 50). Interestingly, mindful people tend to notice their surroundings more, but seem to be less distracted by them, and better maintain focus.

5. Talk to yourself

With practice, you can train your mind to pay attention on command, by literally telling yourself where to focus. Elite cricketers use keywords to focus their attention, saying "ball" to focus on the next shot, "play straight" to put attention on technique and so on. This stops them thinking about themselves, which is the main cause of choking.

Training your attention is hard work. Your mind naturally wanders, so forcing yourself to focus takes effort and it can't be sustained indefinitely. If you are finding it hard to concentrate, don't panic: this is a natural part of how your mind works. Notice what affects your concentration and the times and places that you work best, and make the most of these moments to get more done.

SUPERTASKERS

Psychologists Jason Watson and David Strayer have found people who are brilliant at doing more than one thing at once. They suspect some jobs may have more of these "supertaskers": emergency room doctors, fighter pilots or air traffic controllers might all have an increased capacity to handle multiple tasks. For most of us, though, multitasking is bad for productivity. You might feel like you're getting more done, but you will probably be thinking less clearly, remembering things less accurately and making more mistakes.

MANAGE ENERGY, NOT TIME

One of the most popular areas of productivity literature is time management. Every busy person has, at one time or another, been attracted by the idea that managing time effectively could help them squeeze a few extra drops of time from the day.

The problem with time management is that no matter how good you are at concentration, you can only sustain it for a short while. Eventually, your mind will get tired and your productivity will drop. Time management fails to solve our productivity problems because not all time is equally productive. So the third principle of productivity is to manage energy, not time.

MENTAL ENERGY
Because you can only sustain intensive concentration for short periods, what matters is not how much time you spend on a task, but how much energy you are able to give to it.

In psychology, this is sometimes known as relevance theory. Rather than working through tasks systematically like a computer, your mind is instinctively lazy. It wants to save energy, by prioritizing things according to their relevance: the maximum return for the minimum amount of thought.

This is a smart strategy, because it means you spend your time where it can be most effective. The trouble comes when you try to force yourself to work differently, overriding your mind's natural instincts and trying to work beyond your mental capabilities. This can feel like a good way to get things done, but it can lead to mistakes and problems, and cost you more time in the long run.

Remember, using your conscious mind is tiring. Your thinker uses energy much faster than your sprinter (see page 14), and concentration is a form of mental work that takes energy. When you are tired, it gets harder to be thoughtful, and you are more likely to fall back on old habits, lazy thinking and instinctive reactions. This is fine for simple tasks, but it's no good for complex or analytic work.

To maximize your productivity, then, you have to manage your mental energy, and make sure your mind is in a good state to work effectively. You can point your mind in the right direction, but you won't go far without fuel in the tank.

TIREDNESS AND THE MIND
In 2011, the management psychologist Shai Danziger and his colleagues at the Columbia Business School conducted one of the most influential studies on the importance of managing mental energy. They studied the effects of tiredness on the rulings of judges. A judge's only job is to think things through carefully and fairly. The study, though, found judges would grant parole in approximately two-thirds of cases when their minds were fresh, but nearly zero cases after a few hours without eating or taking time out. Hungry, tired judges were more likely to reject parole requests, regardless of the merits of the cases, because they were too tired to think them through properly.

These and other similar findings have changed the way we think about productivity.

It isn't enough to put in the hours: you also need to keep your mind in good shape to ensure that you can focus on what you are doing.

You can't perform at your peak all the time. Instead, you have to make the most of the times when you feel fresh to get the important things done. Try to make important decisions first, when you have the most energy. If you have a lot of important things to do, don't waste your energy on unimportant tasks; save your mental resources for what really matters.

It isn't always easy to know how tired your mind feels; we all have different clues that tell us when we need to take a break. Think about your physical, mental and emotional energy. How much enthusiasm do you have for this task? Are you able to hold it all in your mind or is it difficult to focus? Are you feeling physically drained or do you feel ready to run a mile? Tune into your mind and train yourself to notice how you feel, or you may not even realize when you're being inefficient.

MAKE TIME FOR YOUR MIND

Don't wait until you're exhausted to take a break, because by that point you've probably already made a few mistakes. Instead, build regular breaks into your routine, taking time out to do things to calm yourself down and wake you up.

Everyone's different, so you need to find the breathers and restorers that work for you – your own personal mindapples (see page 85). Some might be physical, such as going for a walk, others may be more intellectual or emotional. Speaking to a friend, having a laugh, playing a game; all these things can help you reset your mind and get back on track.

RESPECT YOUR RHYTHMS

If you are able to organize your day as you like, think about when it is you do your best work, and prioritize your most difficult tasks for those moments. When you feel tired, do easier things that take less thought.

The goal with productivity is not endless activity, but sustainable engagement. Keep your motivation levels up, but maintain your wellbeing as well. If you work all the time and never take time to rest, very soon you will become less productive than you were previously. In fact, recent studies on overtime show that after a couple of weeks, working more than 50 hours a week actually makes most people less productive.

A CHANGE IS AS GOOD AS A REST

Rest is important, but sometimes what you need is to change, not stop. In his wonderful 1908 self-help book *How to Live on 24 Hours a Day*, the writer Arnold Bennett argued that you can do more with your day if instead of doing nothing when you feel tired, you do something fun instead. Playing tennis, learning a language, practising the violin – all these things can be energizing if you've chosen to do them, and you enjoy them.

LEARN TO SAY NO

Many of us feel overwhelmed by the sheer volume of things that need to be done. One of the biggest sources of stress is having too many tasks and too little time. This is why the fourth principle of productivity is learning to say no.

Saying yes is a habit. Before you can think about a task, your sprinter (see page 14) is already off and running, imagining how you might do it, how long it would take, and so on. This is possibly the wrong approach: it means your mind has already started working on it before you've even decided if it's worth doing. If it's just a time waster, you don't want to spend energy thinking about it.

Productivity isn't just about sprinting ahead: you need to use your thinker (see page 15) too. Whenever you are asked to do something, first think about why you should do it. Ask why the task matters, what the point of it really is. Think about your motivations, the values and incentives that drive you, and ask what would happen if you didn't do it. If there are no serious negative consequences to saying no, then cross it off your list.

WHAT DO YOU WANT TO ACHIEVE?

For the goals you keep on your list, think about the most efficient way to achieve them. If the goal is to get a form filed on time, work back from the deadline and think what is the minimum effort to get that form completed. If your goal is to support your friend, think about how you can show your friend you care, not just

by helping them but also by taking the time to talk to them and see how they are. Focus on what you're trying to achieve and go after it.

PRIORITIZING TASKS

There are various tools for prioritizing tasks. One of the most famous is Pareto's principle, which holds that 80 percent of your productive output comes from 20 percent of your effort. It isn't a scientific ratio of course, but the idea is that if you can identify the portion of your work that has the biggest impact, you can drop most of the rest without losing much productivity.

Another useful tool is Eisenhower's Box, a delightfully named technique attributed to President Eisenhower that involves sorting tasks into their urgency and importance. We do too many urgent things, and not enough important things, says the theory. Unimportant urgencies clog your task list, and stop you from doing things that really matter. Stop doing things just because they're urgent and put your attention on the non-urgent, important tasks.

BE ASSERTIVE

Very often, we say yes to tasks because we don't want to let people down. If you care about other people, as well you should, and particularly if you are high in agreeableness (see page 26), you may find yourself taking on extra work and stresses in order to make life easier for other people.

This is where assertiveness comes in. Resist the urge to martyr yourself. If you want to help your friends and colleagues, then help yourself too. Don't just take on things to be nice: think about where you can add the most value to other people, and prioritize those tasks. Not only will you get more done, you may also find you have better relationships too.

It's difficult to break the habit of saying yes, but doing less is a part of achieving more. In many professions, the difference between the highest performing people isn't what they do, it's what they don't do. In fact, the investor Warren Buffett said that, in his experience, the difference between successful people and very successful people is that very successful people say no to almost everything.

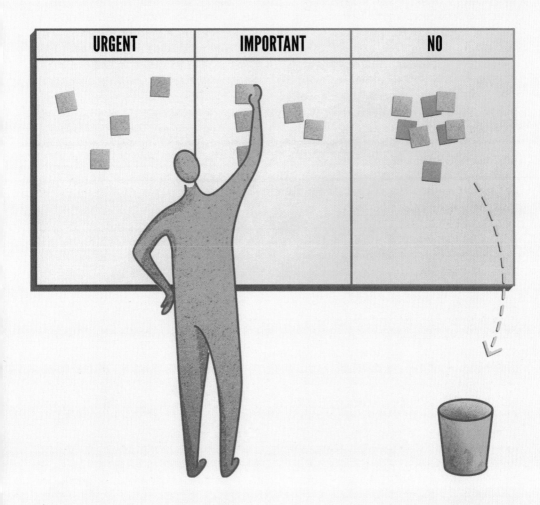

BUILD GOOD HABITS

Not all productivity has to be thoughtful. You have limited attention, but you can get around this bottleneck by learning to do things without thinking.

We run most of our lives on automatic pilot. Your automatic mind, the sprinter (see page 14), is always active, always engaged. Anything that you do regularly, your sprinter remembers how to do it. Practise it enough, and you can do it without thinking – freeing your conscious mind up to be even more productive.

TRAINING YOUR UNCONSCIOUS MIND

The fifth principle of productivity is to build good habits. Your sprinter doesn't care what it learns: it just repeats whatever you give it. You can turn this to your advantage by using your conscious mind to train your unconscious mind. Learning new skills takes work, but once they are automated your mind stores these new patterns so you can do them without needing to concentrate.

Take driving a car, for example. When you learn to drive, you start out slow and ponderous, thinking about each stage consciously, but then with a bit of practice you start to speed up, until eventually you can do it without thinking. This process is known as adaptive learning. Conscious learning leads to unconscious ability.

NEW HABITS

Forming new habits takes a long time. In one 2010 study, students were asked to practise a new habit every day until it was automatic. The average time to reach "maximum automaticity" was 66 days, but some took 18 days, while others were still working on it three months later. Habit forming isn't an exact science.

Think about the skills and behaviours you need to practise, and work toward them. Make time in your week to practise these skills, and after long enough you will find yourself doing them naturally. Try to build your routine to focus on positive habits and avoid negative ones. Otherwise you may end up with a mind that is perfectly adapted to a life you don't want to have. (For more on habits see pages 82–3.)

BRAIN CHANGES

London taxi drivers have to learn The Knowledge, a comprehensive map of every major driving route through central London. They begin by learning each route consciously, but over time, they can do it without thinking. This process physically changes their brains: their hippocampi (small seahorse-shaped parts of the brain involved in memory) grow larger when they learn The Knowledge. When the taxi drivers retire, their hippocampi shrink back down. The brains of musicians show similar adaptations; their brains change as they practise.

TRAIN YOUR MIND

mindapples

FINDING THE BALANCE

Productivity isn't everything. The danger with our modern obsession with efficiency is that we risk doing the wrong things faster. Getting to Inbox Zero isn't much good if it comes at the cost of your health, happiness or relationships.

PRESENT–FUTURE BALANCE

The ever-present spectre of technology is making it easier to work, but harder to stop working. It's tricky to put work to one side when the emails keep coming and the phone keeps ringing. It is no wonder, then, that our obsession with productivity appears to go hand in hand with talk of work–life balance and wellbeing.

Work–life balance is perhaps the wrong term for it though. Work can be meaningful, and many of the tasks that are weighing on your mind may be personal, from sorting out the house to looking after kids. Instead, present–future balance might be a better term, whether you enjoy your life now, or later.

The paradox of productivity is that we work so hard to get more time, and then don't know what to do with the time we've saved. Get things done, make life better for yourself and the people you love, but don't focus so much on the future that you are unable to enjoy the here and now.

SEEK OUT SILENCE

The addiction researcher Stephanie Brown argues that busyness is an addiction, and that we focus on productivity because we are scared to stop. But silence, patience and quiet reflection are a part of productivity too. Slowing down can be agonizing, but maybe we should push back against the cult of productivity.

Silence and stillness are good for our minds. The sheer volume and pace of modern life puts a strain on our concentration, so taking time away from sensory input and doing nothing can be very good for resetting your attention, and can help you concentrate better in the long run. The environmental psychologist Stephen Kaplan at the University of Michigan has even coined a term for it: attention restoration theory, the process by which we recover our capacity to focus.

EMAIL OVERLOAD

Most office workers are drowning in email, and this is one of the most common reasons for low productivity. Tom Stafford of Mind Hacks has argued this is because email is addictive. Every new message provokes uncertainty, because it might be good news, or it might be bad news. Since you never know until you open it, you have to keep checking, just in case. Do this enough, and checking your email becomes automatic.

Silence is good for creativity too. Daydreaming is a key part of the creative process, and making space in your mind can make it easier to think up new ideas, make unusual connections and solve problems. There is even a 2013 study that suggests that periods of silence can help regenerate the brain, rebuilding pathways for learning, memory and emotion.

USE YOUR TIME WISELY

It's hard to stop when the world expects you to be always running though. The pressure to be busy is greater than it's ever been. In fact, complaining about how busy you are can be a way to feel important. If you are constantly overloaded with tasks, then your life must matter. Being pestered by people all the time can be stressful, but it certainly makes you feel useful.

TIME OR MONEY: WHICH IS MORE IMPORTANT?

Worrying about the evils of materialism can be a rich person's game, and the pressures of poverty can be brutal, but it seems the key benefit of wealth is not more money, but more choice. Perhaps the greatest luxury in life is to choose how you spend your time. In fact, one study published in 2016 suggested that people's happiness can be predicted from one key question: whether they value time over money. Those that valued time seemed to be modestly, but predictably, happier.

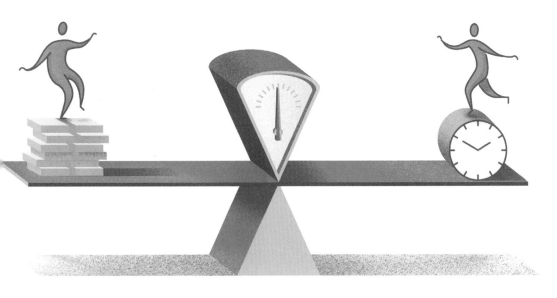

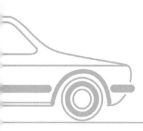

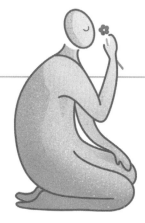

Try not to focus so much on achieving your goals that you miss the unexpected joys along the way.

When we talk about being productive, what we really mean is whether we are progressing toward our goals and achieving our ambitions. Rather than thinking about how many things you've done, think about what you've achieved. Are the things on your to-do list really going to benefit you? Being productive at the wrong things is an efficient way to waste time.

Productivity, like efficiency, is just a means to an end. It's good to save time on tasks, but your goal shouldn't be to have an efficient life, speeding from birth to death as quickly as possible. Life is meant to be unproductive. The inefficiencies tend to be the best bits.

Getting things done takes effort. It is a daily struggle to keep on top of things, stay motivated, focus your mind and get stuff done. Don't waste it. Ask yourself what you're willing to struggle for, and when you have it, enjoy it.

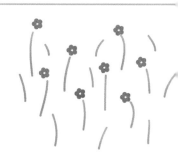

GET TO KNOW YOURSELF

What really motivates you and why?

What helps you concentrate, and how can you make more time to focus on what matters?

Where do you spend your mental energy?

What things can you afford to drop from your to-do list?

How does your routine affect your mind, and are you practising the things you really want to be good at?

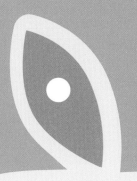

WHAT WORKS FOR YOU?

Make lists.

Create structure for the day.

Respect the sanctity of tea breaks.

Create some clear space between
work and play.

Remind myself how far I've come.

HOW
TO
BE
RESILIENT

HOW TO BE RESILIENT

UNCERTAIN TIMES

There's an old saying in boxing: everybody has a plan until they get punched in the face. It's all very well to have ambitions for your life and good intentions for your heath and happiness, but life may have other plans for you. Sooner or later you will have to deal with setbacks, losses and problems.

Success in life isn't just about how you pursue your personal goals; it's also about how you cope with adversity, and bounce back. Failure and change are just realities of life. The first step is to acknowledge this, and then work on moving forward.

You will hear a lot of people saying that the world is more uncertain than ever. The pace of change, new technologies, the volume of information coming at us, the global nature of modern life: all of these things create pressure on our minds. And yet, if you look back through history, it seems every generation has felt they were facing greater problems than previous generations. Climate change is a threat to us all, but so too was the Black Death. We fix one problem, and another one takes its place.

THE ILLUSION OF CONTROL

The real problem with uncertainty is that it makes us feel like we are not in control. Control is vital for your wellbeing. Having your plans destroyed by forces beyond your reach can feel frustrating and frightening, and it can be tempting to just stop trying. What's the point of making plans if success is out of your hands?

The technical term for this is "locus of control": the extent to which you believe you can control the events that affect you. People with an internal locus of control, who feel they can do things to affect and improve their lives, tend to bounce back from setbacks and feel more positive. People with an external locus of control, who believe their fate is controlled by external forces about which they can do little, are more likely to become stressed and depressed.

You can't control everything though. Life is just too complicated, and there are a lot of other people who want to be in control too. Feeling in control is a matter of perspective. If you have control over the important things, you can cope with uncertainty elsewhere. In fact, we spend a lot of our time pretending that we have more control than we do, comforting ourselves with rituals and superstitions and making neat ten-point lists to explain complicated subjects.

Take travelling by airplane, for example. When you fly, you have almost no control over your safety. And yet, the experience of flying is one of complete control, from the button to summon the flight attendant to the personalized in-flight entertainment, and even the safety card in the back of the seat. All of these things make you feel like you are in control, to distract you from the uncomfortable reality that you are hurtling through the sky inside a metal box.

Life isn't scripted; it is improvised. Make plans and set goals, but also learn to respond to the unexpected. You can't plan for every eventuality, but you can give yourself options, by building your resources and learning from your mistakes. Give up on the illusion of control, and start planning for uncertainty.

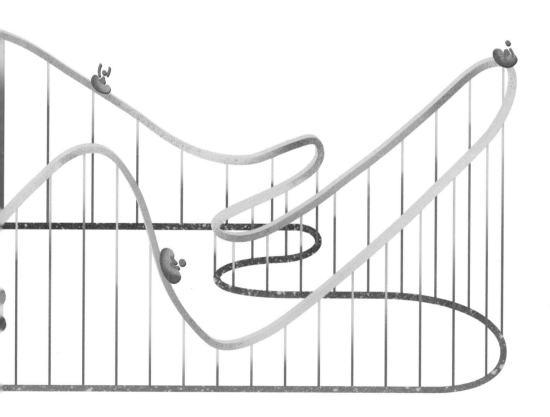

RESILIENCE

Resilience is your capacity to maintain your wellbeing and respond effectively in the face of obstacles and setbacks. It isn't about being insensitive and numbing out your feelings; it's about adapting to stress and change, coping better and bouncing back quicker.

RESILIENCE THEORY

Research into resilience began as an investigation of childhood development and adversity. Rather than studying the negative effects of trauma, the clinical psychologist Norman Garmezy studied what helps some children thrive in difficult circumstances, with the hope of learning what these children were doing right. Since then, the field has flourished into a wider exploration of the habits and qualities that help people of all ages deal with difficulties and setbacks.

Resilience theory holds that, although there are various things that can make you more vulnerable to problems and trauma, there are protective factors that can insulate you from the negative effects of adversity. By managing the risk factors, and developing protective factors, you can become more resilient.

Some of these protective factors relate to the world around you and the support network that you have built for yourself. Good relationships, a safe environment, social support and good education can all help you to bounce back from setbacks. Some are internal to you though, such as how you interpret events or develop positive mental habits to manage negative emotions.

WHAT DOES IT MEAN TO BE RESILIENT?

So is resilience a quality that some people have and others don't, or is it a process that anyone can learn? Bonnie Benard, a specialist in children's resilience, found that resilient children often have four things in common:

- They are good with people, making positive impressions and building lasting, supportive relationships.
- They are good at solving problems, deploying their resources well and asking for help when they need it.
- They have a strong sense of self and confidence in their abilities to take control and succeed at tasks.
- They have a sense of purpose and faith in the future, setting goals, having ambitions and being persistent in pursuing the things they want.

If you have all these things, it's hardly surprising you can cope better.

HOW TO DEVELOP RESILIENCE

How can we turn resilience into a manageable goal that can be practised and refined without the need to turn ourselves into superheroes? At a practical level, resilience is about how you identify and respond to problems. It is a process of awareness and action. Resilience is about asking yourself two simple questions about what's happening:

1 How is this affecting me?
2 What can I do about it?

It's tempting to skip straight to taking action, particularly if you feel stressed or angry, but the first question is hugely important.

Resilience starts with self-awareness, understanding how your mind is being affected by the events in your life. This is about knowing yourself well enough to understand how things affect you, and tuning in to your mind to know how you are feeling at a given time. This process of self-awareness is vital for helping you to respond better. Unless you know how things are affecting you, you won't know how to respond.

We all have different sensitivities and tolerances for setbacks. The people who are most likely to need to develop resilient behaviours are those who are high in sensitivity (see page 22), because they are more likely to be affected by negative life events and emotions. People very high in sensitivity will need to manage their moods and emotions more, and develop better strategies for dealing with adversity. People who are lower in this trait are likely to find it easier to bounce back from problems, though they may also be less able to empathize with the struggles of others.

How can we turn resilience into a manageable goal that can be practised and refined without the need to turn ourselves into superheroes?

Yet resilience isn't a quality we are born with: it is a set of skills and habits that can help you respond better to stress, loss, trauma and the many other obstacles life throws at you. Some of us need to manage our minds more than others, but everyone can benefit from learning positive ways to respond to adversity.

Tall trees grow from strong roots. What can you do to give yourself a stable foundation from which to grow?

HANDLING PRESSURE

We all face pressure at some point. Money worries, family problems, illness, difficulties at work, the constant demands of the modern world...These all affect our peace of mind and threaten our wellbeing.

Handling pressure requires a bit more than your normal coping strategies. As we saw in Chapter 2, too much pressure can make you stressed, your mind's ancient emergency response to fight back or run away (see page 38). Pressure doesn't have to make you stressed though.

Your mind interprets pressure in one of two ways, depending on the resources you have to hand.

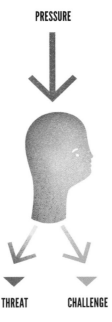

PRESSURE

THREAT   **CHALLENGE**

When you face a pressurized situation, your mind assesses the situation to see whether it is a threat or not. Consciously or unconsciously, you ask yourself one key question: "Do I have the resources to deal with this?"

If you don't feel you have the resources to cope, then the situation will feel like a threat, and you will get stressed. If you do feel you have the resources to deal with it, it will feel like a challenge, and you can actually feel quite excited about it.

Understanding this relationship is the key to handling pressure better. In fact, the stress researcher Stevan Hobfoll has argued that managing stress is all about managing and deploying your resources. Rather than focusing on the amount of pressure you are under, focus on the tools you have to deal with it.

WHAT ARE YOUR RESOURCES?
Anything you rely on to accomplish tasks, solve problems or keep your life running smoothly is a resource. Here are a few examples:

Knowledge and skills
Anything you know how to do yourself is a resource. The things you've learned over your life, the experience you've built up, the skills you've mastered; all of these things can be useful in handling pressure better.

Many new and unfamiliar situations can make us stressed because we don't have the experience we need to handle them. However, having done something, it starts to feel more manageable, until eventually you can handle it without worrying at all. This process of building your skills is a great way to reduce stress.

Confidence

You can have all the skills and resources you need to handle a situation, but if you don't believe in your ability to respond, it can still feel stressful. This is particular to the task: you might have confidence in your memory, but not in your ability to fix a sink; be a confident public speaker, but a nervous date. Confidence is built through experiences of success, trying things out and learning how to do them well. The more you stretch your abilities and take on new challenges, the easier you will find those tasks next time.

Other people

Not all your resources have to belong to you: you can borrow resources from other people or ask for help. Each of us has different skills and expertise to bring to situations, and you can get more done if you know a wide range of people with a diverse set of skills. In fact, most of the complex pressures we face today rely on other people. This can be a source of stress if someone lets you down or creates problems, but generally people are assets. Maintaining good relationships, personally and professionally, will help you handle pressure.

Money

Money isn't everything, but it's certainly useful. Being able to spend more money on solving a problem, or being able to afford to gamble or lose money, can broaden your options and make it easier to deal with pressure.

Money is a tool for getting other people to help you. If you need a hand, and you don't

TURN DOWN THE PRESSURE

Of course, the other way to reduce stress is to reduce the amount of pressure that you are under. It can be tempting to take on more and more challenges but you can end up drowning in pressure and finding no number of resources will ever be enough. If you are really determined to remove stress from your life, you may need to learn to say no (see page 114). Pressure can be fun, but working within your resources is the best way to keep calm and manage those pressures sustainably.

know anyone who can do it, you can pay a stranger to help. Remember though: money isn't the only way to get people to help you.

Tools and technology

One of the best things humans have learned to do is to use tools. We can use objects and props to help us achieve things, and build machines to perform tasks for us. If you have a smartphone, for example, you have half of the world's information in your pocket. Make use of the tools at your disposal, and invest in technology that makes your life easier.

Mental resources

Your mind is your greatest asset. Sometimes you can feel overwhelmed by a task, but then get a good night's sleep and come back to it, and suddenly it feels manageable. Maintaining your mental and physical wellbeing can help you handle pressure better.

RESOURCEFULNESS

The more resources you have, the more likely you are to be able to handle the challenges life throws at you. The challenge of handling pressure, then, is to keep track of the resources you have, and use them to respond effectively.

The difficulty though lies in the fact that stress narrows your focus. When you get stressed, you focus more on the threat and less on opportunities, blinding yourself to your resources and creating a vicious circle of rising stress and lost perspective.

IDENTIFY YOUR RESOURCES

Breaking this vicious circle is fundamental to handling stress effectively. When you are stressed, you need to consciously remind yourself what you are good at, and the people and assets that could help you. Make a list of your strengths, skills and experience, the things you have done in the past and the times when you've overcome problems successfully. Go back through your contacts book and think about who might be able to help you. The more resources you can identify, the more manageable the situation should feel.

It isn't always easy to think about yourself in such a positive way but it is a key part of responding effectively, to break out of stressful fight-or-flight thinking (see page 38). The more stressed you are, the more effort you need to make to broaden your perspective. When you are stressed, you miss things. Keep asking yourself what you've missed. Other people can help you too. Ask friends and family what they think are your key strengths to help you identify assets you might have forgotten. Other people often have a clearer perspective on our troubles than we do ourselves.

BUILD YOUR RESOURCES

Handling pressure is a balancing act. As the pressure increases, you need to increase your resources too. Maintaining a good balance between the challenges you take on and the resources at your disposal is a key part of resilience. Whether you have ambitious goals for your life, or just want to keep calm, building your resources is essential.

A better word to describe this might not be resilience, but resourcefulness. The pressures you face may not be under your control, but the resources you bring to them are. Learning new skills, gaining experience, building supporting relationships and acquiring assets can help you handle more pressure and take on bigger challenges. You can't predict the future, but you can prepare for it.

Don't wait until you're already under pressure to do this. The psychologist Barbara Fredrickson's broaden-and-build theory (see page 64) suggests learning skills and forming new relationships is much harder when you are stressed. The time to develop your resources is in quiet moments, the times when you are less busy and less stressed. Think about what's coming up, and take steps now to prepare yourself for future pressures.

TIPS FOR BEATING STRESS

When the pressure hits though, all these good ideas can go out of the window. The best way to manage stress is to build good habits so you can respond to stress positively, even when you're too stressed to think.

TIPS FOR MANAGING STRESS

Here are three good habits that you can use for handling stress better:

1. Know when you're stressed

Watch for the signs of stress and learn to identify the factors that cause your stress.

2. If you feel stressed, keep asking yourself what you've missed

Write down the problem, talk it through with other people, and map your skills and resources to make overwhelming tasks seem less daunting.

3. Take opportunities to protect and build your resources

Learn new skills and acquire assets to prepare yourself for future pressures.

TIPS FOR SUPPORTING OTHERS

It's hard to think through a problem when you're panicking about it. Sometimes we need help from other people to figure out what to do. If you have a friend or colleague who seems stressed, here are a few things you can do to help them:

1. Find out what matters to them

Ask them why this situation is important to them, and identify the reason why they feel threatened. What are they worried might happen? What do they want to achieve? You never know quite what people are really stressed about until you ask them.

2. Help them spot things they've missed

Stress narrows people's focus (as we saw on pages 40–1), so you need to help them get their perspective back. Ask them to talk you through the situation, explaining each part until they feel more in control.

3. Ask what would help

You are a resource for them, so offer to help if you can. What's more important, though, is to help them think about what help would be useful, to focus their mind on solutions, not on the threat.

Above all, try not to get stuck in stressed ways of thinking. Staying stressed for a long time can affect your mood and make the world seem like a hostile place. Train your mind to see beyond the threat. There's more to the world than pesky tigers (see pages 38–9).

TRAINING YOUR MINDSET

How you feel isn't just about what happens to you; it's about the stories you tell yourself about your experiences, and what you make them mean. You can be outwardly comfortable but feel anxious or depressed, while another person might be experiencing terrible problems but feel positive and full of purpose. You may know what's going on in someone's life, but you don't know what's going on inside their head.

A lot of recent research into resilience has focused on mindset: the explanatory frameworks that you use to make sense of your experiences. Research by the psychologist Carol Dweck and others has shown how people's mindsets can influence their wellbeing and quality of life. Dweck identified two types of mindset as particularly important:

- A FIXED MINDSET: People believe they have fixed abilities and limited options to improve and develop.
- A GROWTH MINDSET: People feel they can change, develop their skills and grow as a person.

THE BENEFITS OF THE GROWTH MINDSET
This subtle difference in mindset seems to make a big difference to how people live and work. In one survey of Fortune 500 companies, fixed-mindset employees tended to be less motivated, less creative, kept more secrets and cut corners to get ahead. Growth-mindset employees, on the other hand, showed more commitment and had more capacity for innovation and ability to manage risk.

The growth mindset's sense of flexibility and possibility can be very helpful in times of difficulty. Feeling that you can change yourself, or change your situation, can make obstacles feel temporary, and give you hope that the future may be different. In fact, having a fixed

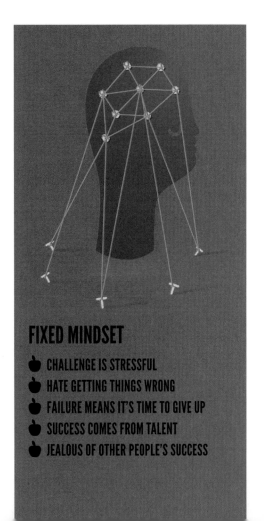

FIXED MINDSET

- CHALLENGE IS STRESSFUL
- HATE GETTING THINGS WRONG
- FAILURE MEANS IT'S TIME TO GIVE UP
- SUCCESS COMES FROM TALENT
- JEALOUS OF OTHER PEOPLE'S SUCCESS

mindset may be more tiring. Hanging onto a sense that things should stay the same in a world that keeps changing is exhausting, using up valuable mental resources that could be better focused on something else.

The statistician and author Nassim Nicholas Taleb calls this capacity to be flexible and handle change "antifragility". The term is mostly used to describe complex systems in physics and engineering, but it can be a useful metaphor for the mind too. It is possible to thrive in adversity, because we can take advantage of a volatile situation to improve and grow. There is evidence that some kinds of failure and setbacks can be positive because they help us develop new skills, learn about ourselves, force us to set ambitious goals and have more compassion for others.

However, with that said, be mindful of not belittling or dismissing someone's hardships as simply an opportunity to build character. Poverty and trauma cause real damage to people's wellbeing and life chances, and this shouldn't be explained away as the result of poor mindset.

A WORD OF WARNING

The danger with this approach, and with resilience in general, is that it can locate the problem in the person rather than the world around them. You are not to blame for feeling bad, so give yourself space to feel sad, angry and upset. Negative emotions are useful, and not to be dismissed as failure or weakness.

Talk of resilience and growth mindsets can sometimes be a way of telling people to shut up, and shaming people for speaking out against injustice. Resilience is important, but it is no substitute for resistance.

The two aren't mutually exclusive though. Learning how to cope in difficult times doesn't stop you from changing things for the better. In fact, a resilient mindset can give you the strength you need to resist more effectively.

GROWTH MINDSET

- LIKE A CHALLENGE
- LEARN FROM MISTAKES
- HARD WORK PAYS OFF
- SUCCESS IS ALL ABOUT EFFORT
- INSPIRED BY OTHER PEOPLE'S SUCCESS

HOW TO BE SAD

Another way we respond to adversity is with sadness, grief and depression. These can rob us of energy and make it harder to take action.

Sadness seems to last longer than other emotions, hanging around, dragging you down and affecting you more and more. In many ways it is the opposite of anger (which we already explored on pages 42–4), a slowing of your system and a flattening of your emotions. People who feel sad even feel physically colder and prefer warmer foods to give them energy.

GRIEF

One of the main causes of sadness is grief, the intense feeling of loss following the death of a loved one or the end of a relationship. Grief is a complex process and takes different forms depending on the circumstances. Sidney Zisook, one of the most influential researchers on grief and bereavement, has observed several different aspects of grief, which can arise at different times for different people:

- **SHOCK: A state of disbelief and avoidance, refusing to accept what has happened or deal with feelings.**
- **SEPARATION: Intense feelings of missing the person, loneliness and helplessness, feeling lost without them and thinking about them.**
- **REGRET: Thinking back to past events and wishing things had been different, feeling guilty or wanting to live things over again.**
- **WITHDRAWAL: Avoiding people and struggling to form new relationships or move on with life.**

Often grief is intense but short-lived, a period of shock and painful emotions mixed with positive memories, fondness and even a sense of needing to live life differently. Grief has a way of waking us up, reminding us that life is short and focusing our minds on what really matters.

In some cases though, it can become a long-term paralysing state, something that must be managed, almost like a disability. Some grief never completely leaves us. Being functional isn't always the same as being healed.

Sadness seems to last longer than other emotions, hanging around, dragging you down and affecting you more and more

---

DEPRESSION

One of the biggest problems with feeling sad is rumination. This is the flip side of worry. Worry is thinking obsessively about future events; rumination is thinking obsessively about the past. When you feel sad, your mind can fixate on the cause of your sadness, thinking about it over and over until you feel sad all the time. Rumination is a problem because it can lead to depression.

Depression is a mood disorder, so it isn't directly related to the events happening in your life right now; it is when sadness becomes part of your inner state, shaping all your reactions and distorting your perspective. If you can't even remember what made you sad, but you still feel flat and lifeless, you may not just be sad: you might be depressed.

Depression isn't simply sadness: it is lifelessness. It suppresses your mind and body and makes it hard to get motivated or do things you need to do. Even pleasurable things can feel impossible. Typical symptoms include loss of appetite, boredom, trouble sleeping, feeling irritable or angry at the world and sometimes physical symptoms such as aches or pains and exhaustion.

Depression is a terrible condition in which life can feel meaningless. You go through the motions, but nothing seems to matter; your home becomes nothing more than a place where you keep furniture; friends feel like strangers who won't leave you alone; even basic actions require a titanic effort.

In some cases, depression can be mixed with periods of manic enthusiasm and an over-

YOU ARE NOT ALONE

Depression is a serious business, but a lot of things can help. So take it seriously, like you would any other health condition and seek professional advice, either for yourself or others. Asking for help is a part of self-help.

active mind – so-called "bipolar" depression, because you can swing from one extreme "pole" to the other. This is a difficult condition and can leave you delirious one day, and in despair the next. This is a particularly high-risk mindset because it makes people more likely to take action to deal with their despair – sometimes with drastic consequences.

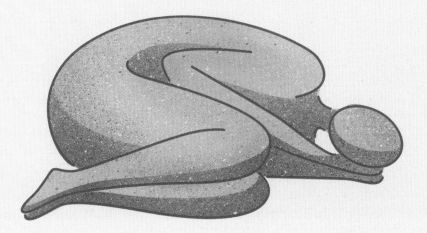

MIND YOUR HEAD

mindapples

ASKING FOR HELP

If you are really struggling with your mind, don't suffer alone. Other people are your resources, and it's really important to ask for help if you feel depressed or overwhelmed.

We aren't always that good at asking for help, particularly with the health of our minds. The temptation is to struggle on and make the best of things. Part of this is due to the huge stigma and fear that surrounds mental illness.

We aren't taught much about our minds, so when something goes wrong the temptation is to think the worst. You don't want to ask for help in case it turns out to be serious. But as with all areas of health and wellness, it's a much better idea to get help early on than wait till things are really bad.

If you are struggling, don't wait until you feel desperate to reach out. Talk to someone as early as you can, ask for advice, and get some insights into how you're feeling. Very often, a little bit of advice or support at the right time can help guide you to the right solution.

If you notice that your mood is low or that you are feeling constantly upset or anxious, talk to someone about it. Speaking to your doctor can be a good start, but so too can speaking to a counsellor or a therapist, going to a peer support group or just talking to friends and family. There are a lot of people around who care, have knowledge and skills you don't, and want to be useful. Give people the opportunity to help you.

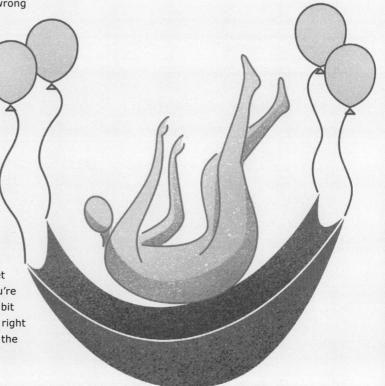

THE JOY OF CARING

The easiest way to deal with adversity is to switch off, disengage from your emotions and say it doesn't matter. This is sometimes what people associate with being resilient: to cope with everything that's thrown at you without feeling bad, or even feeling at all.

And yet, there is a lot more to life than coping. Resilience says little about enjoyment or fun, the people you love or the things that make life worth living. In fact, it is often our attachments to these things that cause us to suffer, mourning the loss of a friend or loved one, or worrying about betraying our principles.

those experiences and learn to live full, meaningful lives.

Perhaps for this reason, many positive psychologists now talk less about resilience and more about self-actualization, fulfilment and flourishing. Resilience is a useful skill, but it is not our end goal. The real goal is to live.

Don't let negative experiences stop you from enjoying life. You can live your life avoiding hardship, but when you look back, it won't be the hardships that you will remember, but the good times, the people you love and the moments you share. So aim for more than just coping: aim to live a full and meaningful life, even if it hurts sometimes.

> ## Aim for more than just coping: aim to live a full and meaningful life, even if it hurts sometimes

Negative emotions and experiences are not an inconvenience to be removed: they show us the things that matter to us and give meaning to our lives. Sometimes we may not even want to feel better, because caring about people and principles can matter more to us than just feeling good in the moment.

ENJOY YOUR LIFE

If being resilient is to mean anything useful, it must include caring about the world, not just enduring it. The goal is not simply to avoid stress or sadness, but to move beyond

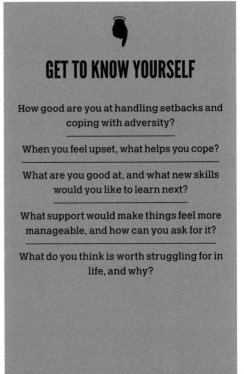

GET TO KNOW YOURSELF

How good are you at handling setbacks and coping with adversity?

When you feel upset, what helps you cope?

What are you good at, and what new skills would you like to learn next?

What support would make things feel more manageable, and how can you ask for it?

What do you think is worth struggling for in life, and why?

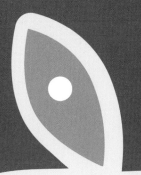

WHAT WORKS FOR YOU?

Accept that things happen for a reason;
even the bad stuff.

Be grateful for what I have.

Daydream – escapism is like a holiday.

Do something outside my comfort zone.

Try to remember that everything
will be relatively OK.

HOW TO BE KIND

KIND MINDS

Despite arguments, intolerance, violence and general stupidity, the backdrop of human civilization is actually one of kindness. For every angry mob smashing the place up, there are millions of other people cleaning up after them, helping out strangers and looking after each other. We have the capacity to be cruel, but we have an even greater capacity to be kind.

THE PRISONER'S DILEMMA

In the 1980s, the political scientist Robert Axelrod studied how people collaborate using the prisoner's dilemma game, in which two people must work together to win, but can also sell each other out. Most people play tit-for-tat, collaborating with people who help them, punishing those who don't. It's a strategy many of us have adopted in our lives: we help our friends, and don't help our enemies.

Yet the results of Axelrod's experiments were surprising. Tit-for-tat works for a while, but it has one fatal flaw: people make mistakes. We betray each other by accident, pressing the wrong button or misunderstanding the rules. We think people have betrayed us when they haven't, and punish them for things they didn't do. Rather than selfish competition, the strategy that works best is being generous and forgiving. We aren't perfect, so we make up for it by being nice.

The process of human evolution seems to be one of increasing cooperation. The early history of our species is peppered with violence, but our story is one of slow progress away from our aggressive roots, toward forming families and societies.

An instinct for compassion may even be as much a necessity for the survival of our species as physical strength or the capacity to use tools. The more altruistic we became as people, the more of us survived, the larger our brains grew and the smarter we became. We won the evolutionary game because we learned to be kind to each other.

> For every angry mob smashing the place up, there are millions of other people cleaning up after them, helping out strangers and looking after each other

KINDNESS IS ITS OWN REWARD

Even if you don't care about being kind to other people, there are good selfish reasons to be selfless. The altruism researcher (and Buddhist monk) Matthieu Ricard has argued that the rewards of generosity are so significant that we need to develop a study of psychological economics that looks past self-interest and measures the rewards that come from helping others.

Volunteering and "giving back" to your community seem to increase wellbeing, and being active in community life can help you feel happier and more satisfied, particularly as you get older. Helping other people even seems to increase life expectancy. In one 2009 study, people who took care of a partner or family member who was unwell were more likely to live longer than those who did not. The pain of seeing a loved one struggling was still distressing, but the act of taking care of them seemed to bring out the best in people and boost their health.

GET THE KINDNESS HABIT

You don't need to give your whole life to community service to feel the benefits of helping others. Try performing one simple act of kindness once a week over a six-week period, and you should feel an effect. Kindness is a habit, so much so that the UK's New Economics Foundation recommended volunteering as one of its five top daily actions for boosting wellbeing.

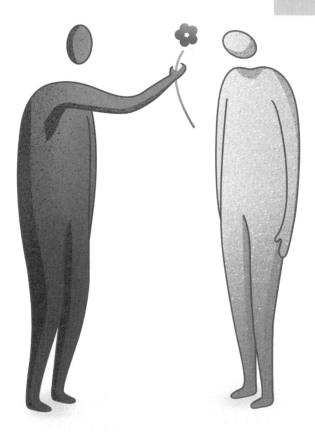

COMPASSION

So important is this human tendency for kindness that in 2008 Stanford University established an entire department to study it. The Center for Compassion and Altruism Research and Education studies altruism, empathy and even morality, and attempts to unlock the scientific code behind our noblest intentions.

While they haven't yet developed a pill to make people nicer, they have discovered some intriguing things about the science of compassion. It seems that compassion comes more easily when we feel safe. If you feel safe you have more headspace to empathize with the plight of others. If you feel threatened, watching someone else suffer can make you feel scared and pull away. To some extent, empathy may be a luxury of the comfortable.

HOW TO BE MORE COMPASSIONATE
Some people do seem to be naturally more compassionate than others though. Highly agreeable people (see pages 26–7) often prioritize the feelings of others more, and put the interests of others before their own. They may also feel more empathy, a greater sense of connection to other people's feelings. But less agreeable people still feel compassion for others, and it is an ability that all of us can learn and improve.

A surprisingly simple (though challenging) method for learning and improving this skill is through compassion meditation, a practice of wishing good things for people and the

world. These exercises help to train your mind to develop kind instincts. There are many different techniques for achieving this, but one of the easiest is to simply look around, wherever you are, pick the nearest person and wish for them to be happy. Small things make a big difference. Even a simple act of imagining what life is like for other people can make you feel more tolerant.

Being kind is a form of pleasure

Surrounding yourself with compassionate people and searching out stories of compassion can help too. Compassion is contagious. The more you see people being kind, the more it inspires this same action in you. Similarly, your compassion will influence those around you.

COMPASSION IS ENJOYABLE

Being kind is actually a form of pleasure. Brain-scanning studies suggest being kind is a similar experience to eating chocolate, and not an unpleasant duty. Even making charitable donations seems to trigger a sense of reward, as if giving to others were a gift to ourselves too.

THE SOCIAL MIND

Part of the reason compassion is so contagious is that emotions and experiences are contagious too. We don't just experience our own emotions; we experience other people's too, physically sharing in each other's happiness.

The set of processes by which this happens is known collectively as emotional contagion: our ability to share moods and converge emotionally with people around us. If people around you are anxious, you will naturally feel a little anxious too; but laugh, and the world laughs with you.

This instinct to tune in is an automatic response – the sprinter, not the thinker (see page 14). You can ignore it, but you can't stop it. People who spend time together often end up sharing moods and emotions. Smiling because a stranger is happy, feeling edgy when someone has a nervous twitch; these responses show up throughout our lives.

MIRRORING EMOTIONS
One of the mechanisms by which this happens is the mirror neuron network. Mirror neurons were first found in the brains of macaque monkeys, by the neuroscientist Giacomo Rizzolatti and his colleagues at the University of Parma. The researchers were studying how monkeys' brains control movement, measuring their brain activity as they picked up peanuts. Then one day, one of the neuroscientists got peckish and ate a peanut himself.

The monkey watched him intently, and to the researchers' great surprise, its neurons fired in just the same pattern as when it had eaten the peanut itself. The act of watching the scientist eating triggered the experience of eating in the monkey's brain. At first this seemed to be a mistake, but it turned out to be a widespread and repeatable phenomenon, and one that occurs in similar ways in our brains too. Whenever you see a person experiencing something, your mind steps through the process, imagining what it might be like – mirroring their experiences.

These responses help us learn skills, mentally rehearsing actions by watching the people around us, and they also seem to play a role in empathy, helping us to imagine what other people are going through and feel connected to their experiences.

TUNING IN TO OTHER PEOPLE
Studies of the neuroscience of communication show that the process is surprisingly physical. The brain patterns of people listening intently seem to track those of the person speaking. We tune into each other mentally and emotionally, giving literal meaning to the phrase "on the same wavelength".

We call this process of tuning in "rapport". When we interact with others, we tend to match their behaviour. If we are with happy people, we laugh and smile more, we breathe faster around anxious people, and so on. All our conversations are full of these unconscious cues, showing each other that we are listening, empathizing, taking an interest. This generally happens without thinking, but you can make a conscious effort to build rapport in lots of ways, some physical and some verbal.

The next time you speak to someone, think about the signals you are giving them. Are you showing them you're paying attention, or thinking about something else? Notice how they are mirroring you too, and adjust your behaviour to show them you are in tune with their state of mind.

Don't overcomplicate it though: when you genuinely pay attention to someone, you will naturally find yourself building rapport with them. If you're too busy thinking about how to show them you're listening, you aren't really listening.

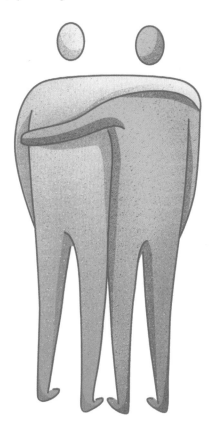

HOW TO BUILD RAPPORT

Here are a few tips to help you build rapport with others:

Make similar gestures and facial expressions to show you're listening.

———

Mirror their energy levels and the speed of their movements.

———

Match their tone of voice and the speed of their speech.

———

Adjust your posture to match theirs and show openness to them.

———

Talk about areas of mutual interest and shared experiences.

———

Repeat what they have said in your own words to show you understand.

THOUGHTFUL COMMUNICATION

Sometimes, just talking to people can feel like a minefield. Many of the difficulties we have communicating stem from the messy use of language. Saying the wrong thing can cause anger, tears and confusion.

Learn to think before you speak. Develop that crucial space between thinking and speaking in which you can consider whether the words you've chosen are right, and the impact they may have on the other person. You can't think things through all the time, but if you want to get your point across, take a little more time to find the right words.

KIND COMMUNICATION

There are many different theories about good communication, each with different things to recommend them. One of the most popular is psychologist and mediator Marshall Rosenberg's non-violent communication. Rosenberg summarized a lot of research into communication to create a sequence for talking to people about what you need in a way that doesn't bully or antagonize them. It can be a useful model to follow when you need to say something cleanly and clearly.

1. Get clear on the facts
State what you know to be true, and focus on the things that everyone agrees happened.

Don't try to interpret them or tell people what they mean to you. Just state the data.

2. Say how you feel
Be personal here: don't talk about the world or other people, just focus on yourself, how you feel, rightly or wrongly. No one will know what's going on in your head unless you tell them.

3. Explain your needs
Talk about why you feel the way you do, what has affected you and how you'd like things to be. This is a chance to be positive, to talk about what success looks like, not about what happened.

4. Make a request
Think carefully about what would help you, or what the other person can do to improve things, and don't be afraid to ask for it – knowing you may not get it. Give people a way to help you.

THE IMPORTANCE OF LISTENING

No form of communication is foolproof. Sometimes you will end up saying the wrong thing or getting your words mixed up. So don't forget to listen too. Ask questions, pay attention to the answers and try to see things from the other person's point of view. Communication is a two-way street you know.

SORRY SEEMS TO BE THE HARDEST WORD

Why is it so difficult to apologize? Saying sorry is such a simple thing, and has such profound effects, so you might think we would do it more often than we do. But apologizing can feel impossible, a threat to our pride or an admission of defeat.

Mistakes happen though, and forgiveness is vital. It is so easy to offend someone, forget a promise, lash out when you're angry, say the wrong thing or otherwise upset people, often without even noticing what you've done. Learning to say "sorry" can be extremely useful.

ACKNOWLEDGE WHEN YOU'RE WRONG

Nobody likes to think they're in the wrong. The experience of being wrong feels exactly the same as being right: the only way you can tell is by listening to others. If lots of people are telling you you're behaving badly, perhaps they have a point. Err on the side of caution: if people want you to say sorry, then say it. What harm can it really do? Many of our problems in relationships come from being so attached to being right, that we forget how to get along.

CHOOSE THE RIGHT TYPE OF APOLOGY

There are many different kinds of apology. Sometimes you need to show remorse and shame for what you've done, to show the other person that you accept their point or agree to do what they asked. Other times you simply need to acknowledge your mistake and put it right. It depends how badly you've behaved and how upset the other person seems to be. Grovelling over a minor issue can look self-indulgent, making the situation all about you, while a cursory apology can seem flippant and make things worse if the incident was serious.

Different sorts of apology are appropriate for different types of people, so you may need to adjust your approach to apologizing depending on the situation:

- If the person you are apologizing to is quite low in agreeableness (see page 26) and less worried about relationships, then focus on making things right. Repair the damage, fix the problem or otherwise compensate them for the issue.
- For more agreeable people, who care more about relationships, then you may need to empathize with their position and show you care. Try to imagine how they must be feeling, and try to repair your relationship.
- If the person you've offended is quite conscientious (see page 24) and likes to follow rules, then you need to acknowledge the rules.

ACCEPT APOLOGIES

Apologizing is a two-way street, and sometimes you will be on the receiving end of an apology. In these situations, it's useful to assume a positive intention, that people aren't malevolent and out to get you. The majority of our problems in relationships are due to honest mistakes. There is even a term for this, Hanlon's razor: the idea that the most likely explanation for people's bad behaviour is incompetence.

Try to see things from the other person's perspective, and imagine what might be going through their mind. You won't always know why people do what they do, but chances are they are also struggling with too much on their plates, reacting badly when they feel tired, stressed or angry, and making stupid mistakes. If you can forgive yourself for being human, you should forgive other people too.

LET GO OF YOUR DIFFERENCES

There may be times when you need to take a stand for something you believe in, and push back against things that you think are unacceptable, but think carefully before putting principles over people. You may be right, but that doesn't mean the other person is entirely wrong. If you focus only on the disagreement between you, you can miss a lot of good things. In the words of the late British politician Jo Cox, "We have far more in common with each other than the things that divide us."

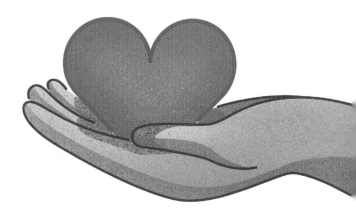

HOW TO HELP PEOPLE

Despite our occasional differences, we usually find it hard to watch someone else suffer. Most of us instinctively feel empathy for someone in pain, and want to help. We look for support when we feel stressed or upset too, seeking out other people to tend and befriend us.

HOW CAN WE SUPPORT EACH OTHER?

Supporting people can be difficult. No one wants to say the wrong thing and make somebody feel worse, and so the temptation is to say nothing, pretend everything's fine and avoid an awkward situation. Sympathy is easy; acting on it is the hard part.

If you have a friend or loved one who is upset, there aren't any magic words that can make things better, but there are a few general principles to follow if you want to support someone effectively:

1. Express sympathy

When someone is feeling bad, a really simple thing to do is acknowledge how they are feeling. If someone is grieving, remember to say how sorry you are for their loss. If they're stressed or panicking, say their situation sounds stressful. It might not sound like much, but it's actually quite important. If you skip over that first step of expressing sympathy for their situation, it can leave them feeling unheard and alone. Say simply and clearly that you are sorry to hear what happened, and then they know you're listening.

2. Ask questions

Questions are more interesting than answers. The best way to engage people in a subject is to ask them a really good question. If you ask people questions, you are giving them an active role in figuring things out; if you only give them answers, they often don't know what to do. Start by asking people what they think, and then share your perspectives with them.

3. Share your experiences, cautiously

When someone shares something that has upset them, the obvious thing is to tell them you have experienced the same thing.

JUST BE THERE

Don't agonize over finding the right words. The first rule of helping people is to show up. Simply being with friends and family can help people recover from trauma, cope with setbacks and find comfort in hard times. Being in good company can calm us down, help us cope and even reduce physical pain. So don't feel you need to fix the problem immediately: just make sure the person knows you're there, and that they can ask for help if they need it. You are being useful even when you're doing nothing.

There is a good intention behind this: by expressing solidarity with that person you can help them feel less alone and show them their feelings are normal. The risk though is that no two experiences are quite the same, so comparing your experience to theirs might make them feel misunderstood or patronized. Secondly, it can take the attention off the person who is upset and onto you, making you seem selfish. Show solidarity, but do it cautiously and keep it short.

4. Put them in control
Beware of solving people's problems for them. The best thing you can do is to show someone how they can solve a problem themselves. Think about how to put them in control. You don't need be silly about this though. If someone asks for your help, help them.

5. Don't pry
While it's helpful for people to talk about their problems, don't feel you need to force them to share. People can have all kinds of reasons for not wanting to share what's on their minds, and often it's because they've hit on something particularly personal or important to them. Aim to create a space in which people feel they can share if they need to, but don't feel pressured to do so.

6. Resist the urge to cheer people up
We all like to spread positive feelings. If someone feels upset, your first instinct may be to try to cheer them up, to look for the positives or tell them things aren't as bad as they think. Humour and light-hearted comments can distract people from their problems. The risk though is that you can

GIVING ADVICE

When someone is struggling, the chances are you will have a lot of suggestions for what they should do or say. The problem is, you may not understand the situation enough, or may be projecting your own experiences onto theirs. We all have different needs and priorities, so what works for you can actually make someone else feel worse. You can do a lot of harm by thinking you know what's good for others.

The best time to give people advice is when they ask for it. If someone asks for help thinking through a problem, or feels so overwhelmed they are happy to take any assistance offered, then you have an opportunity to step up.

give the impression you aren't taking their concerns seriously, or that they shouldn't feel so upset. Give people space to feel bad before you start looking for the good.

MORE THAN WORDS

We naturally tune into each other's emotions, so you can have a big impact on someone just by how you feel yourself. If you think there is nothing you can do, think again.

EMOTIONAL LEADERSHIP

Sometimes the most powerful way to help someone is to bring them out of their distressed state by how you are with them. Even being with someone in total silence can change their emotional state in just a couple of minutes. This process is quite simple, but it takes practice:

1. Read the situation

The first thing you need to do is to read the situation. Expressing your emotions appropriately requires you to understand how someone is feeling, and how your emotions will land with them. If everyone around you is feeling sad, then being quiet and sombre will feel appropriate, whereas excitement or humour may not.

2. Tune in to people

The next step is to tune in to how people are feeling, to show you understand how they feel and feel the same way. You can't bring people with you if you're starting from different places. This isn't about what you say, but more how you say it. Match your posture, movements and speed of speech to theirs and do and say things that show you are listening and understand what's happening.

3. Set the emotional tone

Then, once you are in sync, you can set the emotional tone by expressing your emotions appropriately and leading people into a new state of mind. This could be about slowly speeding up your speech, moving faster or raising your voice to help increase someone's energy, or slowing things down to help them feel calmer. You might want to introduce more positive things, smile or tell a joke, or perhaps you want to bring people back to a serious matter, helping them to engage more with what is distressing them.

Tune into how people are feeling, to show you understand how they feel and feel the same way

---

EXPRESS YOURSELF

To express your emotions appropriately, you need to be able to manage your moods. You can suppress your feelings and act in spite of how you feel (which is known as "surface acting", see page 48), but this is tiring and uses up mental energy. Where possible, really try to be in tune with how other people are feeling until you feel a true connection to their state of mind: it's more honest, more effective and less tiring.

Reading the situation, tuning into people and setting the emotional tone: these techniques sound easy enough, but the trick is to put them all together naturally.

For example, imagine a friend has just narrowly escaped a car accident. They are fine physically, but emotionally quite shaken up. You have a fairly good idea what is going through their mind, so you can guess that they may be fearful and in shock, and they probably want to feel less nervous and more in control.

This helps you understand how to respond. If you laugh it off or try to change the subject, you will give the impression you don't care, and they may respond in turn by becoming even more distressed to show you how bad the situation was. Instead, you need to show that you are listening, so you might build rapport by pacing your responses appropriately, talking faster, matching their gestures and energy levels, and so on.

Once you have matched their state, and are in sync with their emotions, you can then lead them into a calmer state by consciously slowing your breathing, calming your voice and gently shifting your own mood, bringing them with you.

This isn't a set of steps to be followed mechanically though, but an act of empathy, of being with someone and sharing their feelings. Helping people is not a simple matter of being cheerful and dragging people with you: it is only by having empathy for other people, and following their lead first, that you can have a genuine influence on them.

In order to influence people, you need to tune in to how they are feeling.

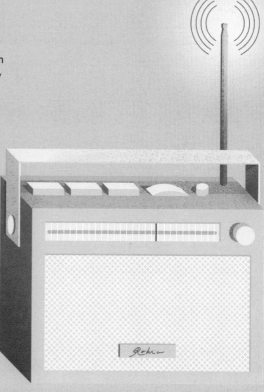

KIND
IN
MIND

mindapples

FIT YOUR OWN MASK

If you spend all your time making sure other people are happy then you may end up with compassion fatigue – too tired to help, and with no energy left for yourself. You can't help anyone if you aren't coping yourself.

AUTONOMY AND RELATIONSHIPS

Life often feels like a balancing act between two basic needs: autonomy and relationships. Autonomy is your desire to be independent and free to choose: it's good to feel that you don't have to do things if you don't want to. However, the need to belong (to a group, a family, a relationship) is powerful too, and we spend a lot of our time doing things to build relationships and bring us closer to other people.

The result is that life can feel like a struggle between these two opposing forces, the need to be independent, and the urge to be interconnected. Individualism is fun for a while, but it sure gets lonely.

And yet, these two basic needs may not be as separate as they look. Recently, psychologists have begun to talk more about relational autonomy, the idea that autonomy comes from good relationships, because other people can help you achieve your goals.

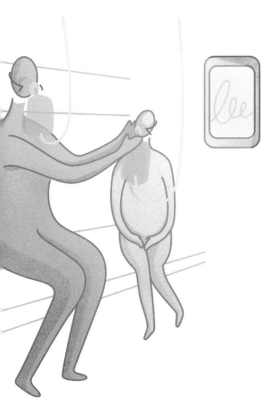

Build yourself a support network of people who can give you the stability you need to be kind to other people

We depend on other people because we choose to, not because we are forced. We put our trust in each other because if we work together we can get more done, have more fulfilling lives and support each other when things go wrong. Selfishness isn't the opposite of altruism; in fact the two go hand in hand.

CULTIVATING SELF-COMPASSION

Being kind means having compassion for yourself too. Self-compassion is a key part of feeling happy and well. Work by the psychologist and self-compassion researcher Kristin Neff and colleagues found that self-compassion was linked to all manner of positive effects, from optimism and positive moods to greater curiosity, extroversion and willpower. It also seems to help people manage nerves and cope with negative emotions. In fact, self-compassion may even make you better at supporting other people.

Neff identifies three parts to self-compassion, each one worth cultivating:

1. Don't judge yourself

Try to accept your flaws and failures like you would accept them in a friend. Compassionate people know that falling short of an ideal is inevitable and you can't always be perfect. Accepting your failures with kindness can help you persevere rather than give up.

2. Remember that you're human

Self-compassion is also about realizing you aren't alone, that other people feel the same way as you, and that you aren't unique or peculiar. Feeling inadequate is part of the human experience, one that we all have to share.

3. Accept your feelings

Rather than getting caught up too strongly in one emotion, learn to notice all your feelings and keep perspective on them. Aim for a mindful, accepting state in which you can feel bad, or feel good, without getting too attached to one or the other. They're all you, and everything is welcome. Don't waste energy suppressing who you are.

CREATE YOUR OWN SUPPORT NETWORK

Above all, make sure you have good support yourself. Build yourself a support network of friends or colleagues who can give you the stability you need to be kind to other people. It can feel a bit self-indulgent to ask for help, but there is no need to be a martyr. Talking things through yourself is part of supporting other people: if you don't look after yourself, you may end up needing the support of the person you're trying to help. As any flight attendant will tell you, always fit your own oxygen mask before helping other passengers with theirs.

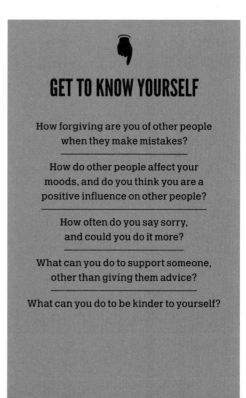

GET TO KNOW YOURSELF

How forgiving are you of other people when they make mistakes?

How do other people affect your moods, and do you think you are a positive influence on other people?

How often do you say sorry, and could you do it more?

What can you do to support someone, other than giving them advice?

What can you do to be kinder to yourself?

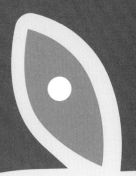

WHAT WORKS FOR YOU?

Talk to people I care about.

Smile at a stranger.

Laugh as often as possible.

Have honest conversations.

Don't take anything personally.

HOW TO FALL IN LOVE

HOW TO FALL IN LOVE

WHY LOVE MATTERS

Love needs little introduction. A million songs have been written about it, people die for it, even kill for it, and we frequently prioritize love over basic needs such as food and safety. Some people even say love is all you need.

For many years, psychologists have been grappling with this elusive but universally human preoccupation. One thing is certain: love matters. Good relationships are essential for our health and wellbeing, and the capacity to form intimate bonds is a key part of positive mental health. Writers such as Sue Gerhardt, a psychoanalytic psychotherapist, have even linked love and affection to basic aspects of brain development, suggesting that when we are starved of love it has a physical impact on our brains.

Good relationships are essential for our health and wellbeing, and the capacity to form intimate bonds is a key part of positive mental health

Yet the way we find love is changing. The commercial juggernaut of online dating is turning the search for love into an algorithm, a streamlined process to find your perfect mate – or at least, someone you think is your perfect mate. Input your desired qualities, click, select and add to cart; then cross your fingers and hope for the best. Finding love in the 21st century can be an alarmingly scientific process.

In this world of ever-expanding options, it's more important than ever to know what you need from a partner, and a relationship. The more choices you have, the more you need to know what you want, where to find it and how to sustain it.

Despite all the time, money and brainpower spent researching love, we don't have a magic formula yet, and it's quite possible we never will. It's hard enough figuring out how one mind works, let alone how two minds can work together. So the starting point for loving well is to think about what love means to you, and the kind of relationship you need.

Is falling in love a science? Despite decades of research and new technologies, how and why we love remains a beautiful mystery.

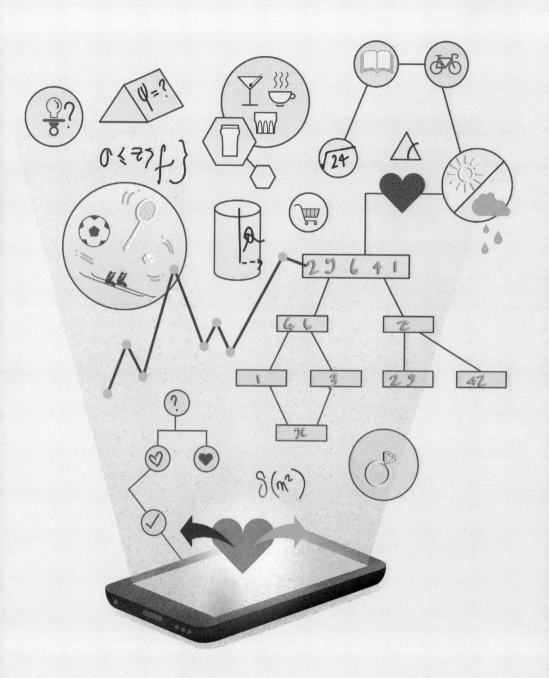

WHAT IS LOVE?

When we hear the word "love", most of us think of romantic relationships. But people also talk about their love for friends and family, their pets, their jobs, homes, holidays, a really good slice of pizza, and even a general love for the world. Love is a word often used, but seldom defined.

So how can one word mean so much? What do we even mean when we talk about love? To help make sense of this, it can be helpful to distinguish, as the social psychologists Ellen Berscheid and Elaine Hatfield have, between two different types of love: passionate love and affectionate love.

Both types of love are "true love", in that they are both measurable in the brain, and both come naturally to (almost) all of us. Passionate love gets most of the attention though. It is what people write songs about, feel despair at losing and place their lives at risk to pursue. Passion usually trumps companionship in modern romantic tales. This may be because watching two people folding laundry together would make for a very boring movie, but it may also be because passion has such powerful physical effects on our brains.

PASSIONATE AND AFFECTIONATE LOVE

Passionate love is like a drug: we experience extreme euphoria and heightened energy levels, and it affects our dopamine systems rather like a stimulant. Like any drug, though, the pleasure is short-lived. Those in search of deeper joys should seek out affection and companionship too. Affectionate love can still involve this rush of energy and reward, but it seems to activate other parts of our brains too, particularly those involved in comfort and family bonding. Romance can be seductive, but coupledom is more complex in its rewards.

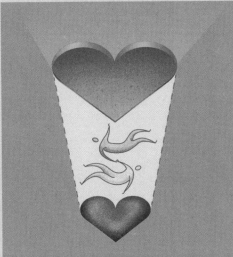

PASSIONATE LOVE

Passionate love is the intense desire for another person. It is a rollercoaster of highs and lows, ecstasy when together and agony when apart. Generosity vies with jealousy, sexual desire lives alongside a need to see their smile. This is the love that you "fall into", and it happens without your control. It might even lead you to ignore the world, or to feel incomplete without the object of your desire. In extreme forms, it can become the obsessive, infatuated love known as "limerence".

WHICH TYPE OF LOVE IS BETTER?

It would be a mistake to rate one type of love over the other. In reality, we need both, and one can provide a platform for the other. Although many couples experience a slowing of intense passion and an increase in companionship over time, affection can lead to passion, and companionship can lead to romance.

Many relationships contain both types, each dominant at different times. You may feel one type of love at one point, and your partner may feel another, which can make relationships complicated. When the "magic" wears off, it is tempting to think you've fallen out of love entirely, but it could just be that your love is changing, and that it could change again in the future too.

This is where our search for love can get a little confusing. We look for passionate love, but end up with companionship, or find passion but can't sustain it when the relationship changes. Some people choose one over the other, and are happy, but the most fulfilling relationships have both.

So if you want to love well, try to nurture both kinds of love. Don't get too bogged down in the technicalities of love though: too much theory can miss the point. The social psychologist and psychoanalyst Erich Fromm considered love not to be a scientific process, but an art. In his book *The Art of Loving*, he writes about love as a creative capacity rather than an emotion, not something to fall into, but to be created together, through care, responsibility, respect and understanding.

Love may not even be a state of mind, but an action, something that you do. In other words, don't wait for love to happen. It's something to go out and create. If you want to be in love, first learn how to love.

AFFECTIONATE LOVE

Affectionate love is a sense of intimacy and companionship, of liking your partner. This type of love burns more gently than its passionate partner, but is no less powerful. This is the love that comes from entwining your life with another person's life, living together, making plans, raising a family, building a life. This is sometimes called Platonic love, but Plato wrote about passion and sexuality too, and affection doesn't have to be asexual. The key is that this sort of love involves a shared focus on the world, not just on each other.

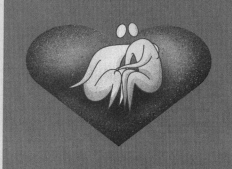

ATTACHMENT STYLES

Just as there are different ways to be in love, so too there are different ways to be in a relationship. We all have different needs and expectations from a partner. For every person who wishes their beloved would never leave, there is another who finds constant contact suffocating.

ATTACHMENT THEORY

One popular model to explain this variation in relationships is attachment theory, which was first proposed by the psychologist and psychoanalyst John Bowlby in the 1970s and 1980s. Bowlby contended that all humans have an innate, evolutionary system that makes us bond with our parents and other close family members in childhood, to keep us safe and provide a stable platform from which to explore the world. We use this same system, so the theory goes, in adult relationships too.

Attachment theory attempts to make sense of our need to bond, and how it varies between people. Some people favour being safe over exploring the world, and others are the opposite. Sometimes our attachment systems can be disrupted by our experiences (absent parents, traumatic relationships) and mix us up. By understanding your attachment style, you can begin to understand the type of relationship that you need, and improve how you relate to people.

CATEGORIES OF ATTACHMENT STYLE

Attachment theory is complex and, like all theories in social psychology, open to interpretation. As always, there is some disagreement about the model among researchers, but there are four broad categories of attachment style that are particularly worth considering.

1. Secure attachment

This is the simplest style of attachment, and the most common. Secure attachment involves being comfortable in a close relationship; being able to commit and make future plans; and finding it easy to enjoy intimacy with a partner.

People who are very secure in their attachments tend to form strong relationships that last. This doesn't mean all of their relationships will be perfect, but it does mean their actions in these relationships will generally be stable and positive. It also means intimate relationships will tend to make them feel safe rather than provoke fear of rejection or betrayal.

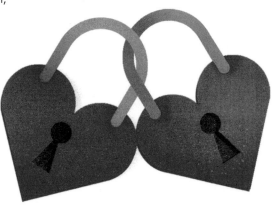

2. Anxious attachment

This style, also known as insecure attachment, involves needing to be in a relationship, fearing being alone and needing regular reassurance to feel safe and loved. Trust can be difficult, and jealousy is common.

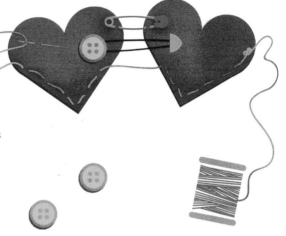

It's still possible to have good relationships with this style, but they are likely to be more intense and dependent. People with this style are more affected by breakups and relationship problems, and two people with this style can even become co-dependent – where both partners are unable to function without each other.

3. Avoidant attachment

Sometimes called anxious-dismissive, this attachment style is also related to feeling anxious in close relationships, but rather than clinging to a partner, people with this style tend to avoid intimacy and commitment altogether.

People with this attachment style may struggle to commit to one person, feel nervous when pressed to make long-term plans, and prefer time away from their partner. It doesn't mean relationships are impossible, but they are likely to be less close and less committed. People with this style are more likely to walk away and feel happier without a relationship. They also seem less affected by breakups.

4. Chaotic attachment

This final attachment style, more commonly called disorganized attachment, involves a combination of the previous two: a strong need to be loved and a strong desire to be independent, particularly to be free from

rejection and betrayal. In extreme forms this attachment style is associated with abusive and unhappy relationships.

People who experience chaotic attachments may miss their partner terribly, but then treat them coldly when they see them. They may resent them for going away, but then walk away themselves – the classic "I hate you, don't leave" pattern. This can be upsetting for both partners, and people with this attachment style tend to struggle the most to form stable, happy, intimate bonds with others.

UNDERSTANDING YOUR
ATTACHMENT STYLE

Attachment theory isn't an exact science: you can't take a quick test and know for sure which style you are, though it might give you some idea. Instead, the best way to think about attachment styles is as a collection of habits that you have developed over the years, learned responses that shape how you respond to people. You won't always feel anxious, or avoidant, or even secure, but over time you may notice patterns in your behaviour, and in your reactions. Understanding how you behave in relationships can be helpful, if perhaps a bit unsettling.

Changing how you respond in relationships is tricky and takes patience – for you and those you love

---

Attachment styles can help you understand other people too, though be careful of labelling people with a particular style – it's impossible to know for sure how someone else experiences a relationship.

If you are anxious in relationships, you may find it difficult to date an avoidant person, who may find you are clingy and not want to give you the reassurances you need. If you are naturally avoidant, you may struggle to commit, feel pressured and need patience and reassurance when taking a big step in a relationship.

Sometimes problems in relationships come because we expect our partners to be just like us, and when they have a different style it can feel like a sign of failure, when it may just be a habit learned elsewhere. Other times, the problems come because we seek people with similar problems to our own, and then blame them when the relationship goes wrong. If you've ever dated someone avoidant in order to avoid having to commit yourself, or blamed your partner for being needy when secretly you like being needed, you have played this game.

CHANGING YOUR
ATTACHMENT STYLE

Attachment styles aren't as rigid as personality traits, and they can be changed. Some studies suggest that 20–30 percent of us change our attachment styles over time, and these patterns seem to be learned rather than inherent. Nevertheless, as with any habit, changing how you respond in relationships is tricky and takes patience – for you, and for those you love.

This is one of the main areas of focus for psychotherapy. There are many different approaches to therapy but a consistent ingredient of therapeutic treatment is the relationship between the client and the therapist. This relationship works like any other, and is therefore subject to all the same patterns and problems as other close relationships – which gives people a chance to explore how they respond in relationships, understand those patterns and work to change them. Very often, the value of the therapy isn't so much what is said, but the process of learning to relate to someone in a healthier and more trusting way.

MIND YOUR LOVE

mindapples

CHOOSING THE RIGHT PERSON

Just as there isn't one single pattern to a good relationship, there also isn't a template for choosing a partner. The "right person" is different for each of us.

SEEKING PERFECTION

Some people believe everyone has one special person waiting for them. It's a comforting idea at first glance, but it gets less comforting when you consider it in more detail. Suppose you never meet? Or worse, you met them and didn't notice? What if they married someone else instead of waiting for you? Given how many things can go wrong in the quest for love, the idea that we only get one shot can be frightening – and it can be destructive too, because you may pass up a chance with someone amazing while you wait for the "perfect" person who never arrives.

The more challenging idea is that there isn't a perfect person for you, but that you have a series of opportunities to build a relationship that works. Rather than thinking about the kind of person you want to be with, think about the life you want, and look for someone who wants the same things as you.

WHAT ARE YOU LOOKING FOR?

Choosing a partner isn't easy. For a start, much of it can feel out of your control: attraction can happen if you like it or not, and you can't force yourself to love someone. Exercising rational judgment doesn't work for such an emotional matter. Falling in love is the domain of the sprinter, not the thinker (see page 14).

The result of this is that we tend to make a few predictable mistakes in our choices. One is the "halo effect": the tendency to think someone is perfect on the basis of one feature. You like someone's voice, and so they must be clever too; they have a nice face, so they must be a nice person. The reality can be dispiriting.

We also exhibit the same familiarity bias that affects all our decisions: people who look like us, sound like us or remind us of our friends and family, all grab our attention and make us feel drawn to them. You can also dismiss people based on surface details rather than giving them a chance. You can't control your initial attraction, but you can avoid reinforcing bad intuitions with false conclusions.

So what should you be looking for? There isn't an obvious formula to what makes a good partner, but there are some patterns.

PERSONALITY TRAITS

In Chapter 1 we looked at the Big Five personality traits: extroversion, sensitivity, conscientiousness, agreeableness and openness (see page 19). These traits can help you understand how a person will react, what they might enjoy and how they fit with your personality. Someone very similar to you will share your comfort zone, enjoy similar activities and want a similar kind of life.

Opposites can attract though, and sometimes you might be drawn to someone who complements your personality. If you are an introvert, an extrovert partner can help bring you out of yourself; someone more conscientious than you can bring a little order to your life. There are degrees to this of course: too much difference and you can find yourself arguing over the washing up, or feeling lonely at home while your partner goes partying. But a little difference can add spice to a relationship, and your partner may shift your personality over time too.

Get to know your comfort zone, and consider the personality traits of the people you choose to be with, and who chooses you. It helps to learn what drives you crazy in others too. If messiness bothers you, date conscientious people; if you are sensitive to criticism, you need someone high in agreeableness. With so much variation in personalities out there, it's no wonder we all fall for different people.

ATTACHMENT STYLES

Attachment styles don't map easily onto personality traits and are worth considering separately (see page 164). People with secure attachment styles tend to build longer-lasting relationships, so if you are anxious or avoidant it can be good to be with someone secure. If you are quite anxious, dating someone else with a similar style can lead to co-dependence, so try to keep up other interests and don't lose yourself. If you tend to avoid commitment and intimacy, dating someone very anxious could be frustrating for both of you.

KNOW YOURSELF

You can't apply any of these principles if you don't know what you need. Perhaps the biggest mistake we make when choosing a partner is that we don't take the time to really get to know people and find out whether their needs match ours. You can feel passion for a stranger, but to form a relationship, you need shared values and similar goals. If you don't understand yourself or your partner, it's hard to know what the future holds.

The best way to attract someone who wants the same life as you is to live that life. Do things you love, keep meeting new people, and don't put up with things that make you miserable. The right person will find you eventually. The real trick is not to mess it up when they do.

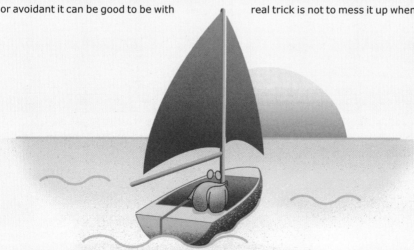

STAYING TOGETHER

It can be tempting to think the hard work stops once you've found the right person, but relationships are an ongoing process, and they take effort.

THE KEYS TO A SUCCESSFUL RELATIONSHIP
Few of us go into a relationship thinking it will fail, and yet we know the majority of relationships won't last. So what are the ingredients for a happy long-term relationship?

1. Passion and affection
Neuroscience findings in 2011 showed that couples who remained in love over many years maintained the same passionate neural responses, alongside those characteristics of affection and companionship. They still wanted their partners, and had a stronger and richer sense of liking them too. Passionate love (see page 162) may come and go in a relationship, but if it is bolstered by sustained affection, it can flourish in the long term.

2. Communication
Lack of communication is often cited as the reason for breakups, but it is difficult to say what this means in reality. Does the lack of communication cause the break down in the relationship, or is it a symptom of when things are going badly? Whichever it is, focus on being clear on what you mean. Very often, arguments are caused not by disagreement, but by a lack of understanding.

3. Trust
Relationships are rather like teams: you need to know the other person is committed to the same goal. Being loyal to your partner doesn't mean telling them every tiny detail, but it does mean taking their interests into account in every decision you make. If you begin to doubt that your partner has your interests at heart, it can cause things to unravel. In extreme situations, this can even affect how much you like them. You may still feel passionate love – you still want them – but, if you don't like them, the affectionate love can collapse.

4. Conscientiousness
Another thing that seems to help make relationships last is conscientiousness (see page 24). If both partners are high in this trait, and capable of controlling their impulses,

PREDICTING SUCCESS

The relationship psychologist John Gottman's research into romantic couples produced an interesting observation. In his opinion, which came to prominence in writer Malcolm Gladwell's 1996 book *Blink*, the most important factor predicting whether a couple will break up is contempt. Relationships in which people show contempt for their partners, criticizing or looking down on them, tend not to last long. In other words, relationships work if you genuinely like your partner – the essence of affectionate love.

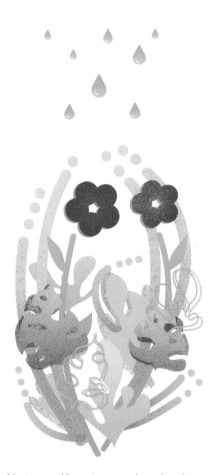

LOVE WILL CHANGE AND GROW

Don't be tempted to freeze the moment. Relationships change, and that's OK. In fact, that's the point. How you feel about your partner now may not be the same five years from now, and how they feel about you will change too. Not allowing people to grow and change can actually be quite harmful. Relationships aren't a fixed point, but a process of moving in the same direction.

The word we give to this capacity to be ourselves with someone else is intimacy. Intimacy is being yourself and feeling completely accepted by another person. Obviously there are degrees to this – everyone needs a little privacy – but generally this experience of dropping our guard and feeling appreciated and understood is vitally important to (almost) all of us. Couples that are intimate tend to like each other more, and want each other more too, even over the long term.

working toward long-term goals and making adjustments for each other, this seems to result in happier and more long-lasting relationships.

BE YOURSELF

Successful relationships are ones that enable you to be yourself. In fact, there is some evidence that in the most successful relationships, each partner incorporates the other into their sense of self, seeing their partner as an extension of themselves.

WORK AT IT

There are a great many pressures on modern relationships. Family tensions, money worries, work pressures, jealousy, disagreements on where and how to live – all couples go through difficult periods. What makes things last is a shared commitment to making things work even when it's hard. It isn't about gritting your teeth, but enjoying being together enough to make the effort worthwhile.

BREAKING UP
IS HARD TO DO

One of the toughest parts of being in a relationship is knowing when to walk away. How do you know when enough is enough?

As should be clear by now, this is not a scientific question: you need to decide what you want, and what you're prepared to tolerate. You need to weigh up your situation now with how you'd be on your own, and not just in the short term, but in the long term too. Breaking up is usually painful and difficult, so you need to know there is something better on the horizon if you're going to make a change.

> ## You might be able to influence how someone feels, but you can't force that person to love you

The best reason to split up, obviously, is if you are unhappy. The trouble is, we aren't very good at knowing how happy we are. As we saw in Chapter 3 (see page 54), we get used to things and struggle to remember how we felt previously. You might think you are unhappy now, but be careful not to romanticize the past or fantasize about a perfect future.

Couples do have irreconcilable differences though. Maybe you no longer trust your partner, or like them as a person. Maybe they want such different things to you that you must choose between being with them and getting the life you want. Maybe you just don't feel anything for them anymore, or worse still, have strong feelings for someone else. Whatever it is, generally you will know when you feel ready to leave. Don't force it: life is short, but not so short that there isn't time to try to work things out with someone you love.

ENDING A RELATIONSHIP

Breaking up with someone requires clarity and sensitivity, often at a time when you feel upset. It's best done face-to-face rather than ghosting (withdrawing from all communication without explanation) or texting. Remember that a great deal of emotional communication is non-verbal, so don't close yourself off: take a deep breath and show the other person that you care about them. Be clear about what you want, explain how things are for you, and ask them how things have been for them too.

Of course, it won't always be you initiating the breakup. Getting dumped is a particularly nasty experience, because it doesn't just mean the end of the relationship, but can also feel like an attack on your self-worth and sense of control. Most people say their relationship is the most important thing in their lives, so when it is taken away it can feel destabilizing and maddening. Our extreme reactions to breakups are in part a response to this feeling of powerlessness.

DEALING WITH JEALOUSY

One of the biggest issues we face in breakups is jealousy. How deeply you feel jealousy will usually depend on your attachment style (see page 164). People who are anxious in relationships may focus their fears on jealousy and fear of abandonment, and look for reassurance. Someone with a more avoidant style may feel less afraid, and instead respond to feeling jealous by withdrawing, or even seeking out someone new.

Some people are able to get over jealousy – even feel happy when the person they love finds joy with someone else – but for most of us jealousy sucks, and it needs to be managed.

It's hard to avoid feeling jealous in a world of constant social connection, but if you do find yourself obsessively checking your ex's

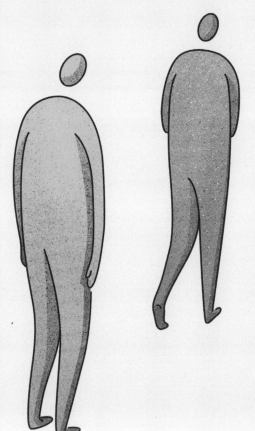

Instagram feed, for example, try to break the habit quickly. Focus on something else, preferably something positive in your life. Managing jealousy is mostly about managing your feelings. Many of the weird, obsessive and destructive things we do, in and out of relationships, are just about managing anxiety or avoiding sadness.

You may also need to manage the temptation to take back control. Control is, for the most part, an illusion. You might be able to influence how someone feels, but you can't force that person to love you. Accepting the things you can't control, and focusing your attention on things you can, is an important part of staying psychologically healthy

DON'T TAKE THINGS PERSONALLY

It is tempting to blame yourself when a relationship goes wrong. It can be comforting to think that there was something you could have done, a simple trick that would have made it all work. However, the trouble with relationships is that there is another person involved too. It's all very well finding someone you love, and treating them well, but the relationship won't work if they don't love you or if they treat you badly. You may think that you can hold a relationship together on your own, but the frustration – and the joy – of a relationship is that it takes two people to make it work.

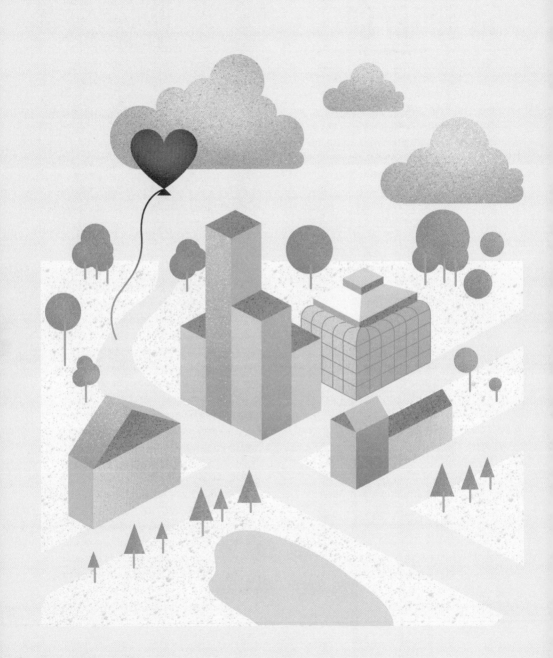

HOW TO LET GO

The end of a relationship is a loss. People may not take your loss seriously, because no one has died and nothing outwardly awful has happened, but people respond to breakups like any other loss, grieving over what's gone and sometimes feeling stuck ruminating on the past.

How you respond to a breakup will be influenced by your attachment style (see page 164) and personality (see page 19). If you have an anxious attachment style, you may feel deeply affected by the end of a relationship, particularly if you didn't initiate it yourself and feel abandoned. This will be amplified if you are sensitive to negative experiences, or if you are high in agreeableness and relationships are very important to you. Someone more avoidant or less sensitive may feel less hurt, while chaotic attachment can make things very confusing, flipping between indifference and heartbreak, and perhaps leading to on-off relationships.

Gender may play a part too: a 2015 study at Binghampton University found that women tend to be more upset than men at the start of a breakup, but recover quicker in the long run.

LETTING GO OF PASSION
What causes these feelings of love and loss to dissipate? In her work on passion and infatuation, the psychologist Dorothy Tennov proposed three ways that intense feelings of love and lust subside:

IS LOVE WORTH THE HEARTBREAK?

The neuroethicist Brian Earp at Oxford University has speculated that drugs could cure us of love, just like any other chemical process. This might feel like an appealing idea in the throes of a break up, but perhaps we shouldn't be too keen to turn love into a scientific process. As Earp himself points out, suffering is a part of how we learn and grow, and we shouldn't be too quick to pathologize it.

- **CONSUMMATION:** Sometimes, the feelings naturally subside the more time you spend with the person, until they become just another person to you.
- **STARVATION:** An alternative (which is not always self-imposed) is that no contact at all with the person can cause those feelings to wane too.
- **TRANSFERENCE:** A third approach is to transfer your feelings of affection and desire to someone else, and forget the other person, which can help in the short term, but sets up potential problems in the future.

WHAT ABOUT AFFECTION?
Affectionate love (see page 162) may not be felt with the same desperate intensity as passion, but it can trigger a deeper sense of loss and grief. This seems to be particularly true if the relationship was close and altered you as a person. If you feel your partner is an extension of your sense of self, losing them can damage

your self-image, and may make you doubt who you are. If they have really hurt you, you may even start hating yourself for their actions.

LOVE AND HATE

This brings us to one of the oldest observations in psychology, that there is a thin line between love and hate. Love and hate are not opposites: they feed each other.

Love-hate relationships involve passionate love without affectionate love. You want them, but you don't like them. The passion you feel for them can even make this dislike more intense, turning minor issues you might ignore in someone else into something huge and terrible in your eyes.

The trouble is, hatred is an intense experience, and leaves very little room for anything else. Disliking someone is fine, but obsessing over the negative aspects of a person is a strangely intimate exercise. Dreaming of vengeance can be satisfying but it isn't very effective. Getting even can be fun, but it won't actually improve your life very much. Perhaps this is why people say that the best revenge is to live well. So try not to obsess over someone you dislike, because it takes up a lot of time and energy that could be better spent improving your life. As the singer Rodriguez used to say, hatred is far too powerful an emotion to waste on someone you don't really like.

Suffering for someone you love is part of being human though, and just because something ends, it doesn't mean it wasn't worthwhile. Getting hurt is a risk worth running in order to find something wonderful. As the old saying goes, everyone is going to hurt you; you've just got to find someone worth suffering for.

GET TO KNOW YOURSELF

Do you prefer passion or affection?

What sort of attachment style do you think you might have, and why?

Who are you attracted to, and how similar are they to you?

What do you think makes a relationship last?

What helps you let go of old relationships, and focus on someone new?

WHAT WORKS FOR YOU?

Tell someone I love them.

Write poetry.

Hug my partner.

Feel our unborn baby kick.

Miss someone.

CONCLUSION

The human mind is one of the most remarkable systems in nature, and each of us has been put in charge of one.

The processing power of your mind is superior to the smartest machine we can build, and its functionality so broad that we can barely map all the things it can do. Your mind can imagine the future, remember the past, construct logical arguments and make sophisticated plans. It has functions to keep you safe, remember people, learn new skills and solve problems. As far as lifestyle technology goes, your mind is still where it's at.

The trouble is, we take our minds for granted. We leave them running all the time, forget to have them serviced, bash them around on our travels and don't recharge them as often as we should. We leave lots of apps running in the background, draining the battery, and we become impatient when they don't do what we want them to do. Like a faithful old laptop, or your first smartphone, you've had your mind for so long now, you've probably forgotten how amazing it is.

IMPROVING YOUR MIND

The growing interest in how our minds work, in psychology and neuroscience, wellbeing and mental health, is encouraging though. Perhaps one day we will genuinely take care of our minds like we do our bodies. We may even see the moment soon where taking care of your mind becomes the norm, and taking your mind for granted is seen as similar to being unfit, not taking care of yourself.

Despite the brilliance of our minds, there is certainly room for improvement too. We can end up slaves to our cravings, doing stupid things and wishing we'd reacted differently, been more considerate or made more effort. Our minds can't be programmed like computers, and because of that, it can feel like we are wrestling with imperfect tools, struggling to be brilliant in spite of our humble origins.

The more we learn about how our minds work, the more tempting it can be to want to improve them. We are capable of great wisdom and insight, but so too of folly, ignorance and predictable mistakes. Our desire for short-term gains might make sense most of the time, but it is little use in averting the impending climate crisis. Our loyalty to friends and family is admirable, until it turns to hatred of outsiders.

So how can we improve our minds, make ourselves smarter and improve our personalities? You can of course take care of yourself, practise good habits, train your attention and compassion, learn knowledge and skills, and manage your emotions. You can build good support networks too, extending your abilities to achieve more, and helping you when you need a friendly shoulder to cry on. As we have seen throughout this book, there are many ways to get more from your mind.

FUTURE POSSIBILITIES

These techniques can only take you so far though, and some people want more radical solutions. One of the more intriguing questions about our minds is how far we might be able to upgrade them in the future. From neural implants to smart drugs, there are people all over the world now working on tools to make us cleverer and calmer. The technology is still in its infancy, but it is coming.

In 2014, the *Wall Street Journal* said brain implants were at a similar stage now to where laser eye surgery was a few decades ago. We can already build neural implants to allow patients simple control over replacement limbs by thinking about movement. Scientists recently boasted technology that could transfer thoughts from one mind to another purely via neural implants. There are too many risks and costs to make these tools worthwhile for most of us, but it is only a matter of time before the technology catches up, and upgrading your brain becomes a serious possibility, or even a marketing opportunity.

Perhaps it will be a drink to boost your mental energy and make you less prone to unconscious bias. Or maybe it will be an implant that senses your stress and calms your mind down, allowing you to respond more thoughtfully in a crisis. One day we could see plug-ins to learn particular skills, like calculating complex probabilities or

playing the Goldberg Variations on the piano. We might even see the creation of technology to increase our empathy for others, allowing world leaders to understand the pain of their people, or helping us see things from another person's point of view.

If this all sounds terrifying to you, then you are in good company. The possibility of upgrading and augmenting our minds is one of the most alarming areas of scientific ethics. Upgrading ourselves is fraught with philosophical dilemmas.

Consider, for example, the economic implications of some people being able to afford to enhance their abilities while others can't. And what if you don't want to put things in your brain, and like your mind as it is – will you be left behind?

Most of all, the possibility of changing your mind begs the question, who are you anyway? If you are the sort of person who worries about your relationships, and then suddenly you are not, then are you still you? When do you stop being the best version of yourself you can be, and become a new version of someone else?

LEARN TO LOVE YOUR MIND

We must hope that this new drive to improve our minds, to stay mentally fit and to be the best version of ourselves we can be, doesn't turn into shaming people who feel mentally unwell, or punishing ourselves for our many imperfections.

Chasing perfection, as the comedian and film producer Steven Wright once put it, is like trying to take a close-up photo of the horizon. Maybe your mind isn't as brilliant as you might like. Maybe you aren't as smart as your colleague, or as calm as your neighbour.

Perhaps you wish you were slightly better at singing, or had more willpower for sticking to your diet. But you are still brilliant. For all our flaws, our minds are remarkable things, and there is much more to celebrate about them than there is to change.

Good mental health isn't about constantly trying to change yourself, it's about learning to live with yourself. Rather than trying to tame your mind, make friends with it. Whether it's trying to keep you safe from imaginary tigers, or nudging you to have more fun, your mind is only trying to be helpful. Don't suppress it. It is part of who you are.

The lesson from all the many suggestions from the Mindapples community over the years, the people who share their mindapples, the participants in our training sessions, the many voices campaigning for better mental health and wellbeing around the world, is that there isn't a perfect way to feel, or a right set of things to do. Our minds are not like livers or kidneys: they aren't just functional; they are personal, and looking after them must be personal too.

So learn to love your mind, and find a way to live in it that feels comfortable and allows you to enjoy your life, be kind to others and achieve your goals. It's about finding your own journey to mental health.

AT HOME IN YOUR HEAD

Ultimately, there is no more private and important space in the world than your own mind. This is where you spend your life, and it is where you return to whatever happens around you. You mind is your home. Clean it, take care of it, dust it once in a while, add an extension if you must. But make sure you enjoy it.

Each of us has to find our own way home. You can follow someone else's path to health, wealth and happiness, but then you will end up living their life, not yours.

So don't try to have the perfect mind, try to have your own mind. The goal of life isn't about being perfect. It's about feeling at home in your head. Because once you have that, the rest of life's challenges will start to feel a bit more manageable.

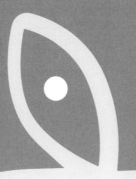

WHAT WORKS FOR ME...

Walk in cities.

Play the piano badly.

Do something I'm good at.

Be myself with people.

Give in to temptation at least once a day.

Andy
X

NOTES

LOVE
YOUR
MIND

mind*pples

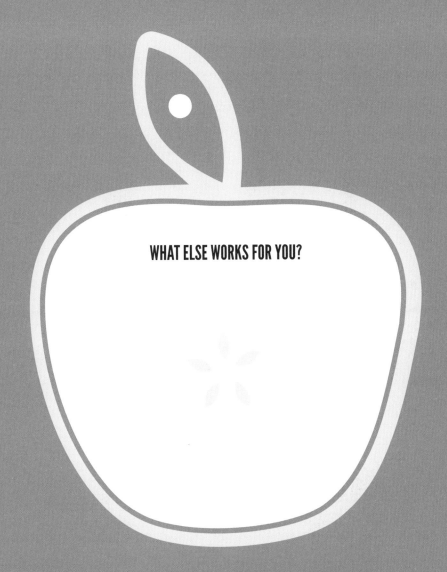

WHAT ELSE WORKS FOR YOU?

What else have you noticed about your mind from reading this book?
Have you noticed any new things that are good for your mind?

Take a moment now to write your five mindapples again, and then
compare them with the ones you wrote on page 9. There's always
room for more mindapples.

INDEX

FURTHER READING

There's a lot of research behind this book, all far too extensive to list here. If you are interested in learning more about the hundreds of theories and research studies upon which this book is based, you can find a full list of references at:

www.andygibson.org/ the-mind-manual

ACKNOWLEDGEMENTS

This book marks ten years since I first had the idea for Mindapples, and so it offers the perfect opportunity to thank the many, many people who have helped it grow.

First, there are the people who helped turn the idea into an organization: Jo Worsley who inspired me to start it, Tessy Britton who persuaded me to do it, Tom Ten Thij, Lauren Currie, Ana Garcia and Kris Morris who planted our first seedlings, Hege Saebjornsen who helped me found the organization, and the gang of friends and volunteers who surrounded the project in its early days.

Then there's Esther King, who worked tirelessly to build the organization with me, and Mindapplers past and present, Ruta Marcinkus, Jenny Reina, Gianna Goulding, Nicola Bonnick Caldeira, Penny King, Hen Norton, Renato Lopes, Laura Yates, Helena Ambrosio, Tanya Hunter, Bryony Timms, Nina Burrowes, Colin Tate, Dan Kolodziej (the bad apple), Sorcha Piotrowski, Rachel Statham, Alex Lucy, Shiraya Adani, and of course Michele Worden, without whom Mindapples would have withered while I wrote this book.

Thanks also to all the people who helped create the training that inspired this book, particularly Ruta Marcinkus, Natalie Nahai, Alex Fradera and Sam Spedding for their help with the content, Amanda Walderman, Anna Golowski, Jana Stefanovska and Desiree Ashton for teaching it to people, Owen Tozer for his epic designs, Unboxed Consulting, Gospelware and Comms Learning for their digital skills, and PB Graphics for being the best print company ever.

Many others have played their part too, from our amazing Headboard, Natalie Banner, David Gold, Patrick Watt (our loyal disc'apple), Richard Armes, Robbie Cowbury and James Glover, to advisers and supporters like Ollie Smith, Kumar Jacob, Billy Dann, Laura Roling, Martin Webber, Alex Murdoch, Lucy Smith, Tony Coggins, Maureen Rice, David Matthews, Eileen Sugrue, Darren Guy, Rohit Kumar, Rich Crozier, Krushma Makwana, Ariam Asghedom, Marjorie Thompson, Paul Mitchell, Nicky Forsythe, Delphine Reynaud, Martin Coyd, Anna Hatton, Chris Oglethorpe, Jenny Rolfe, Jane Barker, Ann Paul, Sarah Jones, Lizz Brocklesby, Mark Williamson, Rebecca Alexander, Paul Farmer, Tim Rawe, Andy Smithyman, Adam Gee, Jamie Hancox, Shane Carmichael, Christine Hartland, and many, many more. I'm sorry if I've forgotten anyone. It takes a lot of cooks to bake a mindapple pie this big.

Which brings us to this book. Thank you to the wonderful Sarah Ford for commissioning it, and the amazing team who made it better than I could have imagined: Polly Poulter, Jaz Bahra, Clare Churly, Jane Birch, Peter Hunt, and of course Abigail Read for her mind-nourishing illustrations. Thanks too to the people who supported my mind while I wrote it: my parents Peter and Sylvia, aunt and uncle Paul and Julia, friends Colin, John, Bex, Roger, Lolita, Michael, Charlie, James, Jon, Ben, Peter, Ofordi, Vanessa, Liz, the Rhombus, and above all my superwife Shanan, who put up with me writing it, read every word of it, and whose feedback was always wise and kind.

But most of all, Mindapples has always been about the volunteers, the friends and supporters who have made us so much more than an organization. We can't do everything, and it's been our loyal gardeners, too numerous and wonderful to mention here, who have really brought our message to the world.

So this is for you. If you've shared your mindapples, asked others to do the same, volunteered for us, bought our toolkits, run events, attended our training, shared our content, or in any way encouraged people to look after their minds, then this book exists because of you. When you have a new idea, it's very hard to know if you are really on to something, or if you've just lost your mind. It is the people who come to help who let you know you aren't crazy. Thank you very much for that.

Andy Gibson
Head Gardener, Mindapples